30 POUNDS
in
40 DAYS

*One Man's Weight Loss Journey
with the HCG Diet, and a
Guide to Losing Weight Fast,
While Creating Lasting Changes in Life,
Health, Motivation, and Habits*

ERIC STODDARD

ISBN: 0990365719
ISBN 13: 9780990365716
Library of Congress Control Number: 2014910026
Createspace Independent Publishing Platform
North Charleston, South Carolina

DISCLAIMER

THIS BOOK IS INTENDED as general information about the author's experiences and not as a medical manual. All information included is for educational purposes only and is not intended to diagnose or treat a disease or illness, to serve as medical advice, as a substitute for medical treatment, as legal advice, or to make any claims. The FDA has not determined that HCG (human chorionic gonadotropin) causes better weight loss than normal exercise and dieting. Before beginning any lifestyle change, such as a diet, consult with your physician. The information given here is designed to help you make informed decisions about your health. The information presented in this book is in no way intended as medical advice or as a substitute for medical counseling. The information should be used in conjunction with the guidance and care of your physician. Consult your physician before beginning any weight loss or nutritional program. Your physician should be aware of all medical conditions that you may have as well as the medications and supplements you are taking.

This book is not written or reviewed by any medical organization and should not be construed as medical advice or
diagnosis of any kind. The information presented should
not be interpreted as a substitute for physical consultation,
evaluation, or treatment. You are urged and advised to seek
the advice of a physician before beginning any weight loss
effort or regimen. This information is not meant to replace
the advice of any physician. Do not rely upon any information to replace consultations or advice received by qualified
health professionals regarding your own specific situation.
Any information provided in this book should NEVER be
construed as medical advice. If you have any question in
your mind regarding any lingering health concern, you
should seek medical advice from your physician.

The information in this book is distributed on an "as-is"
basis, without warranty. The author does not make any
warranties about the completeness, reliability or accuracy
of this information. Any action you take upon the information presented in this work is strictly at your own risk.
The author is not and will not be liable for any losses and/
or damages in connection with the use of this work or information provided. The author shall not have any liability
to any person or entity with respect to any loss or damage
caused or alleged to be caused directly or indirectly by the
information contained in this book.

retrieval systems, without written permission from the author.

ISBN: 978-0-9903657-1-6

To my family: Ken, Shirley, and Andrea,
who have always believed I would write
and who finally convinced me to believe it, too.

CONTENTS

**I lost 30 pounds in under 40 days,
and I did not gain it back.**

While following this plan, I was able to create lasting change in my life and my health, by using specific techniques that I've described in this book.

I offer the perspective of the patient – not the doctor – a regular guy who was actually successful in following his nutritionist's advice, losing 30 pounds in under 40 days, sustaining the weight loss for months, while making permanent improvements in my habits and in my life (not to mention, my clothes now fit much better)! In the over 300 pages that follow, I'll share everything I possibly can about how I made that happen.

More than that, I'll share advice about behavioral change that goes far beyond weight loss. You can apply this advice to any area that requires you to change your habits, from personal finance to your education and even to your career!

Why This Book is For You

This book is about behavior, not medicine.
It's about how to *make* a plan work, not about why the plan could work if executed perfectly.

This book is not written from a doctor's point of view, but rather from a patient's point of view.
This is not about what's going on in your bloodstream; it's about how to actually get the right things into the bloodstream!

This book is written from the point of view of someone who actually made it work!
I was overweight and feeling terrible, and I made massive change occur in a short time period, with sustained success.

The advice in this book can supplement any plan you arrive at with your doctor or nutritionist.
Many books can give you the perfect plan; this book gives you the tools to make your plan work!

This book recognizes that we are not perfect!
I'm a regular person – a human being who makes mistakes, and who isn't usually able to follow any instruction perfectly and consistently. You, like me, are probably a regular person. Most of the advice we read seems to be for *perfect* people – people who never make mistakes. We often hear advice for people who can instantly adjust their diet, completely avoid temptation, clear their schedules to exercise, and have the discipline to do all of this perfectly all the

time. The problem is, almost nobody can do that! Unless you're an elite full-time athlete or an actor spending all day prepping for your next movie role, you don't have the time or focus to make that happen. This book recognizes that we are regular people! We work. We go to school. We do things like eat ice cream with our kids, have dinners out on Saturday nights, and go on vacation. We are busy, and we are far from perfect. This book assumes you are *you* and that "you" do not happen to be infallible.

This book is about behavior, not about rationale.
How many times have you heard a financial expert talk about interest rates on credit cards, when everyone knows the real problem is the fact that people spend too much? It's the same with our nutrition. We hear advice all day long about the right foods to eat and the right exercise to do, when the real problem is that we give in to temptations, binge on terrible foods, and never make time to exercise. The reason for our weight gain isn't because we haven't yet found the perfect kind of organic kale! There's a time and place for theory, and this isn't it! Instead, we'll focus on changing your life habits in the short term, in order to rebuild habits in the long term, translating into lasting change that will ripple through your behavior for years to come.

If you're even thinking about starting *any* plan to lose weight, including an HCG diet plan, this book can help you with:

- Overcoming self-destructive patterns that may have ruined your results in previous attempts to lose weight

- Using your knowledge of your own patterns to plan ahead and prepare to make good decisions

- Dealing with the bad influences around you, like your unhealthy friends who bring cupcakes to work or don't seem supportive when you try repeatedly to lose weight

- Controlling hunger, cravings, and binges

- Eating foods you choose and therefore enjoy, without having to drink some strange, special juice or smoothie every day (unless you want to do that, which, if recommended by your nutritionist, is fine with me)

- Preparing to start your transformation, ensuring you're truly ready to create lasting change

- Teaching yourself to cook, and finding time to make healthy foods you enjoy, even in your busy life

- Opening up to your friends and relatives about what you're doing, and making sure you're set up to succeed before you embark on your transformation

- Selecting the right doctor and nutritionist to get you started and hold you accountable

- Going on vacation without ruining your entire transformation

- Using technology like your tablet, smartphone, Mac, or PC to easily track your weight loss, water intake, and daily nutrition

- Creating visual aids to track your progress and keep you motivated

- Maintaining your weight once you reach your goal, and feeling more in control than ever about maintaining a weight you're happy with for the rest of your life

- Rewarding yourself so that you have something to look forward to

- Creating sustainable, repeatable systems, like creating an "autopilot," so you experience lasting change and don't gain it all back

- Getting used to adding some vegetables into your meals in ways that will make you crave the foods you prepare (think omelets, stuffed peppers, fajitas, and lettuce wraps!)

- Preparing food more than you do now, but finding time to do it, while actually enjoying the process, maybe even with a glass of wine

- Giving yourself a makeover (guys, no makeup required – just some new jeans and maybe a sweater or two) to reward yourself

- Journaling your efforts and progress

What's Not in This Book

THIS BOOK DOES NOT include a comprehensive, step-by-step weight loss plan. If you're looking for someone to tell you, step-by-step, what diet or what plan will work for you based on sound principles of fitness and nutrition, you are fortunate that there are literally thousands of incredible books available to you, written by experts who have studied and researched the subject a lot more than me, and even lost a lot more weight than me over time! Having said that, it's my guess that you've already read one or two of those (if not more), and another perfect diet plan is *not* what you need, and that's where this book comes into play.

In my experience, I've found that many of us have already read countless books like that and are in need of something else. *The book you're reading right now is that something else!*

This book actually started out as a journal I kept while losing weight, and it's meant to be a *companion* to any weight loss plan you choose. Like I've mentioned, I'm a real human being who actually made weight loss work, while dealing with a full schedule of life, work, family, vacations, holidays (I did this weight loss plan through Thanksgiving!), challenges, and even while completing a master's degree. Through all of this, I was able to succeed in changing my weight and my habits, and I believe that the absurd and sometimes inappropriate real-life tools I created to get through this could be helpful to you.

I'm not an expert in nutrition or fitness, and I'm certainly not claiming to be.

As I've mentioned, there are thousands of authors out there who are experts in these fields, and I strongly encourage you to absorb the wealth of information they can provide you through books, websites, blogs, videos, and lectures!

What I offer here instead is the story of my own bumpy road to sustained weight loss. I'm a regular, working guy who spends all day in an office, and spends nights and weekends as a graduate student – my *real* expertise is in typing quickly and showing up promptly to meetings. Even though I'm not an expert in health, fitness, or nutrition, I was successful in a journey that managed to change my life – I want to offer you my story and the set of discoveries I made along the way, in hopes that they can help you change your life and ultimately unlock a little of your hidden potential, in the way that I believe I have.

In this book, I'm going to include everything I did, from the good to the bad to the very ugly. I'll share my strengths, my weaknesses, my thoughts, and my feelings. Whether it helps you to lose weight and create lasting change or gives you a laugh (or both), I am happy to be sharing it with you.

I've included research to back the concepts presented here, but not everything in this book would be recommended by an expert! Experts might even comment that some of the actions I took may even have had detrimental effects! Part of this writing is to entertain you and to show you how I, a normal, imperfect person, couldn't succeed in a traditional, "fix your whole life at once" kind of way but found a way to do it that worked for me. Part of this is to show you that this actually worked and to guide you through your fears about attempting to lose weight, including any fears you may have about the HCG diet (which I used, as prescribed by doctor and nutritionist), by showing you a real human being's example of a journey through all of this.

I won't focus only on the HCG diet here.

Though I used the HCG protocol, I won't necessarily promote it here, nor will I tell you not to use it. I'll give you the ins and outs of what I did, as well as a general overview of HCG's history and the theories around its use. The strategies I used and what I relay to you here can be used with or without HCG, and I encourage you to check out the content of this book whether or not you're open to using an HCG program.

Get a Pen

You'll find that much of this advice can be applied to your life right away, and some of it may not work for you. That's fine! Take notes as you go! Starting now, if you're using a Kindle, use the highlighting feature to create a list of the best ideas you can glean from your reading. If you're reading the good old fashioned paperback version of the book, I suggest you use a highlighter and that you take notes of tips that apply to you as you go. However you read this book, by the time you reach the final page, you'll have a massive list of ideas for how you can apply this advice to your life and your transformation.

For Those With A Lot of Weight to Lose

I want to add a final introductory note, for those of you who have a lot of weight to lose. I certainly don't want to overpromise and under-deliver here, so I'll say this up front. I was someone who was floating at about 40-50 pounds over my desired bodyweight when I started this transformation. If you're someone who has more weight than that to lose, I believe this book can be helpful to you, but you may not relate to the experience I've had, because the situations I'm presenting aren't written by someone who has walked a day in your shoes. The book is geared toward folks who would be very happy with a short-term transformation that most likely equates to thirty to forty pounds of weight loss. I welcome you to read its content and glean what you can, but because this book is based on my personal experience, I cannot say that I've written something here that presents an understanding of what you may have gone through, or the way you may plan to change.

FOREWORD

"You'll gain it all back."

IT'S WHAT EVERYONE SAID, even my closest friends. I was the heaviest I'd been in my entire life, and, like many times before, I had set out to lose the weight. Then, something remarkable happened. I proceeded to lose 30 pounds in under 40 days[1], and I did not "gain it all back!" (To be very precise, I lost 29.1 pounds in 38 days, but titling a book 29.1 in 38 just doesn't work well.) Aside from minor fluctuations since then, I have not gained any of it back, and I've actually lost *even more*.

Let me say this again so it sets in:

I lost 30 pounds in under 40 days, and I did not gain it back.

I lost the weight while following a program that was prescribed for me by my doctor and nutritionist, which included the use of HCG (which I'll explain later). While following this plan, I was able to create lasting change in my life and my health, by using specific techniques that I've described in this book.

I'm not a doctor, I'm not a nutritionist, I'm not an elite athlete, and I'm not a personal trainer. I'm a regular person, probably a lot like you, who has always struggled to maintain a healthy weight, eat healthy foods, and stay fit, in the midst of all of the challenges and temptations that are everywhere around me.

So, why would I write a *book* about weight loss? Like so many of us, I spent every day juggling all the stresses of a busy life, yet I was able to lose 30 pounds in a short amount of time.

I want to tell you that it's possible, and I want to share with you, how I was able to do it.

Perhaps you can relate to where I was before my weight loss. I found myself overweight, struggling to keep up with a high-pressure job, finding no time to focus on my own health or nutrition, with the pounds continuing to pile on. I thought, *How did I get here?* I often thought, *I was meant to do so much more – why don't I have the drive or energy to do it? Why am I just getting by?* In the months leading up to my ultimate point of frustration and, then, my weight loss, I asked these questions more and more. I think we all have.

I believe we hold ourselves back when we aren't in the right physiological state to do what we were put on this planet to do. Said more plainly, I believe we may let ourselves get too unhealthy to think effectively, and too under-confident and tired to do what we really ought to be doing. It's tough to make the contribution you want to make to this world when you're weighed down by your mind, which is being weighed down by your health. I want to show you how I fixed that in my life and how it made a massive change to my productivity and happiness, in hope that my journey may inspire a similar path for you and that you might unlock something in yourself that lets you accomplish everything you want in life and everything you didn't think you could ever achieve!

Why is this book any different from others?

So many books out there seem to be written for people who have the discipline to adhere to a restrictive an unpleasant diet for months. Who can really do that? I certainly couldn't just read advice in a book and follow it! I'd cheat!

This book is for *regular* people, like you and me, who struggle with finding that kind of discipline and who need to find ways to overcome that so that we can live healthy lives.

I think that if an elite athlete or strict vegan were to read this book, he or she would get a laugh out of many of my suggestions, because it sometimes takes every ounce of my creativity and strength to do the things that those people do out of habit every day! If you're like me – someone who just can't always seem to eat what he knows is right, and who has gained weight because of it – this book is for you.

This book contains a wealth of information about a plan based on "HCG" (which I'll describe in more detail later), but it isn't just an "HCG book" or even a "weight loss" book.

This is a guide and a recollection of my journey that includes advice on making lasting, transformative changes in behavior.

I've done plenty of reading about health, fitness, and weight loss, and it has always seemed to me like most books are focused on following ideal behaviors in order to get results. The authors outline picture-perfect step-by-step plans. They include the science behind the plans and the reasons why certain activities and diets work. We need these books and I think we're very fortunate to live in a time when such a wealth of information is easily accessible all around us. Having said that, what many books and plans seem to leave out is what I consider to be the most important part of my recent transformation: *how to get regular people to actually follow the advice!*

So much content is focused on *what* to do, without much (if any) advice on what to *stop* doing and how to stop doing it! We've all been told the reasons to stop doing things (I know I *shouldn't* eat a whole cake right before bed), but we often don't have any clue of how to get ourselves to actually stop doing them! (Why is there cake all over my bed?) The advice that's available all around us often neglects the fact that we, the patients, are not superhuman! We are real people with real lives, unending obligations, and very real bad habits that have been formed over (literally) a lifetime!

When I first visited my doctor and asked him what program I should follow to lose weight, his answer was simple: "Choose whatever plan you want, as long as you're able to follow it."

There's brilliance in that statement.

**Regardless of the plan we choose,
the most important factor is our ability
to actually *follow that plan*.**

In this book, I will demonstrate that my success was
due in part to having a good plan, but also to developing
techniques that enabled me to follow that plan.

INTRODUCTION TO MY
PERSONAL TRANSFORMATION

Me: Before

On November 14, 2013, I was the unhealthiest I had been in my life. When I looked at myself in the mirror, I was unrecognizably overweight. My face was big and round, and my clothes were tight. I could barely fit into anything. I was sluggish and tired. I was under-confident. It seemed like life was not going well.

Me: One Month Later

By December 17, only one month later, I fit into clothes I would not have been able to wear since college, my blood pressure was at an all-time low, and I went from a happy-hour-attending, pizza-eating sloth to a vegetable-eating, exercising, happy man.

Me: Now

Today, months later, my tastes have changed so that I look forward to healthier foods, and I drink less alcohol. During my weight loss phase, I did not exercise at all – I actually relaxed more than I had before! After my weight loss phase, I participated in a half-marathon, for which I barely had to train, because I was so much lighter than I'd been before! (This isn't surprising – according to a recent study published in *Marathon Journal*, runners who lose 10 pounds of weight experience 15% fewer injuries while improving their race times by 22%).[2]

I not only run faster, but I now have a whole new wardrobe, a newfound confidence, and a bigger smile. I hop out of bed faster than I ever have, ready to face the world. Life is amazing! As you know, I've even published my first book!

I'm so excited about what I've accomplished and the new doors that have been opened in my life that I want to share this experience with you, so that you might benefit from what I've learned.

Don't let the title of this book make you think it's only about short-term change. "30 in 40" describes the initial part of this journey, and if you're excited about weight loss, that's great! In the end, I found that the short weight loss period was the smallest segment in the transformation and that the lasting change was far more rewarding. Yes, the weight loss happened, and yes, that's exciting, but most of what I'm sharing here is about making changes that will last forever. Research published in *Obesity and Health* indicates that successful, long term weight loss and maintenance needs to include elements of a paradigm shift within oneself – not just for weight loss, but for a healthy lifestyle.[3] Through this process, I achieved that paradigm shift, and my whole world improved!

The process was about more than just eating the right foods – it was about getting to know myself and establishing habits that would carry me into and through the future, at the weight at which I wanted to be for the rest of my life. Should you choose to do what I did, you may lose weight (I can't guarantee it or even recommend it, because I'm not your doctor), but more importantly, you will know yourself much better and you will establish systems and habits that can make you successful in the long run.

This book is about giving you the tools you need to make a successful lifestyle change and preserve that change. Research published in the *Journal of Consulting and Clinical Psychology* shows that learning a set of "stability skills" before losing weight improves long-term weight management. According to the research, stability skills are designed to optimize individuals' current satisfaction with lifestyle and self-regulatory habits while requiring the minimum effort and attention necessary, and learning these skills before losing weight can be helpful in the long-term maintenance of weight loss.[4] In this book, I'll provide you with the stability skills I learned, and help you to think of ways to create your own.

Sitting here, many months after the start of this journey, having already helped some others to get started on this path, I realize that this program has been more about developing mentally than physically. The reason I've been successful has a lot more to do with what I did up in my head than it does with the food I ate (and did not eat). The eating and the eventual workouts were simply a result of the changes I was able to make mentally, and I was able to make those mental changes using a set of techniques that made me successful. In this book, I'll talk about all of the ways I got myself to a better place, both physically and mentally.

I look at this book as a journey on which I'm going to accompany you, and my goals for our journey together are as follows:

- I want you to realize that losing weight fast while developing habits to keep it off for good is not impossible, and that with the right guidance and mindset, you can actually do it!

- I want to be your companion as you think about going down this path, and I want to give you a virtual "shoulder to lean on" as you think about doing this.

- I want to let you know about the ways I learned to cope with life during this process, and how I spent time understanding my habits and shaping my behaviors to limit the impact of the bad habits, because that's what ultimately led to my success.

- I want to give you the best advice I've got. I'll share every tip that's in my brain, that I use every day to help me to continue my progress. I'll share with you all of the little tricks that worked for me, like buying a ton of food storage containers, drinking San Pellegrino instead of sodas and energy drinks, and making all sorts of foods to "trick myself" into getting vegetables into my system.

- I want to tell you what *didn't* work, like going on a cruise, trying to lose weight when I wasn't ready, and deviating from my plan.

Most importantly, I want to write all of this down for both of our sakes. I want to make sure I have something on paper that I can look back on when times are hard for me. And in turn, I want to share my story with you, so that I might help you to make this happen in your life, and so that we might get a few of those "you'll gain it all back" people to eat their own words and join us, achieving our highest potential, in better health.

I believe that beneath every person who feels overweight lies untapped potential and confidence that will not come out until the weight is gone. I believe that you can make the changes you want to your physique, but more importantly, that your newfound health can help you unlock other dreams that you won't even let yourself have. I believe that you need to be in better physical condition, so that you can think big, and do what you were put here on this planet to do! I want to *unlock you, and* along the way, I want you to be able to wear your favorite jeans again!

Follow me through this. Let me be your bad and good example, and let's meet on the other side – skinnier, happier, healthier, and inspired to dream big!

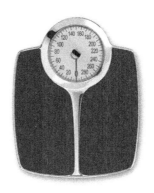

PART 1:
KNOW THYSELF

IF YOU GIVE A MOUSE
A COOKIE...

IF I CAN GIVE you one piece of advice that you can use to improve any area of your life, it is this:

Know Thyself

There's a fantastic children's book you may have read called *If You Give a Mouse a Cookie.*[5] "If you give a mouse a cookie," the author writes, "he's going to ask for a glass of milk." Then, when you give the mouse the glass of milk, he asks for something else, which leads to something else, which leads to all sorts of mouse-related mayhem.

The moral of the story is *one thing leads to another.* If you were this mouse, giving you a cookie may lead to you asking for a glass of milk. Or, and possibly more realistically, giving you a cookie may lead to you asking for another cookie and another cookie and then a whole box of cookies.

Not unlike the mouse's pattern, if you give Eric (me) a Coors Light, he's probably going to ask for another Coors Light. And, if you give Eric another Coors Light, he's going to ask for another Coors Light. If you give Eric yet another Coors Light, he's going to ask you for a pizza. This is just how it works.

Would a completely sober version of Eric ever make a deliberate, informed decision to drink this many Coors Lights and then follow it up with a pizza? No. He would not. But an Eric who has already had two Coors Lights is very likely to make a decision to have a third. And an Eric who has already had three Coors Lights would be happy to order a fourth. Finally, an Eric who has had four Coors Lights will definitely want a pizza and will call to have it delivered. By that time, discipline for the night will be lost, and Eric will wake up the next morning two pounds heavier.

It doesn't need to be this way. I found that in many different areas of my life, by avoiding that first step in the chain of events, I could avoid negative behaviors, and direct myself down a whole new path. During my weight loss, I decided that I was going to *truly know myself*. I was going to know my own habits inside and out, so that I could use those habits in battle with my own mind and to win my transformation.

I *know* that I will drink a Coors Light if I've already had a Coors Light. So, following this example, I used that knowledge to overcome my bad habit. I simply found ways to avoid situations where I would have an opportunity to do the wrong thing. The work of the noted psychologist B.F. Skinner included the concept of "stimulus avoidance," or staying away from certain external factors that affect your behavior, as a strategy for self-control.[6] In line with this concept, during the most intense portion of my weight loss, if people were headed out to a happy hour, I would not join. Why tempt myself? The completely sober, rational version of me would not allow that to happen. I would go home, turn on *The Biggest Loser* or a movie, and just relax. If I felt productive, I would catch up on some email or write a paper (I was enrolled in school at the time). If I felt completely lazy, I would just sit and watch TV, but this was *much* better for me than hanging around influences who would support the chain reaction mentioned above.

From this, I arrived at this key piece of advice:

Knowing yourself inside and out, so well that you can predict your counter-productive behaviors, so that you can then take steps to avoid those behaviors, gives you a tremendous advantage when it comes to weight loss and everything else.

This became the key to my success.

WHY THIS BOOK WORKS, WHEN OTHERS MAY NOT HAVE

LET'S BE HONEST WITH ourselves for a moment. You and I both know enough about nutrition and exercise to lose weight. We've read the advice, we've seen the advice, but we've just never been able to follow through on the advice. We know what foods are good, if you ask us. We know what exercises are healthy.

Our issue is not a knowledge issue, but a behavioral one.

What most of us do not know is *how* to eat the right foods and do the exercises instead of repeating the destructive patterns that guide us every day of our lives.

Our problem isn't that we don't know what to feed ourselves, it's that we've developed bad habits over the course of a lifetime that cause us to not feed ourselves the right stuff and do the exercises we know are good for us.

It's not the wrong plan that's killing us, it's that we can't seem to follow any plan that we try!

If your veterinarian tells you that your pet is overweight and you need to put Sparky on a diet, is it difficult for you? It's probably very easy. It's not hard to only fill Sparky's bowl to a certain line, and it's easy to give him a different kind of food. So, if that's so easy, why can't we do the same for ourselves? You already know the answer. When Sparky begs for scraps, you say, "No!" When *you* beg for "scraps" (or an extra piece of pizza, or a can of cola, or a candy bar, or a whole cake), you don't always say no. (You never say no.)

You probably know *exactly* what to eat and do to lose some weight and be healthier. You just can't make yourself do it.

Follow just about any diet out there, and you'll lose weight. But here's the key to the last sentence: "follow" is hard to do. You can buy any book, watch any video, and talk to any expert, but if you can't find ways to get yourself to follow the advice you're getting, then you're going to fail before you even start.

So why does every book on the shelf seem to be about something new to *do*, and why does it seem like none of them tell you how to make yourself do it?

I laugh to myself as I write this, because it's hard sometimes for us to find the commitment or willpower to even read an entire book in the first place! That being the case, how could we expect to follow the advice in the book for weeks, months, and then for the rest of our lives?

Why would we even *expect* to be able to do this? People out there are recovering from heart disease that stemmed from smoking or a poor diet, yet even *they* refuse to change their habits after doctors have saved their lives! In fact, according to a poll by the Canadian Heart and Stroke Foundation, more than half of heart attack and stroke survivors who needed to make healthy lifestyle changes "couldn't maintain the change and others didn't try at all!"[7] If these people won't change in the face of death, why would you expect *you* to change while you're able to sit upright, walk around, and read this book? Yet every time you lift a diet book or say you'll head to the gym tomorrow, you're expecting yourself to just start doing things differently!

Let's stop trying four to five different diets per year and failing each time (ABC News reported in 2012 that dieters typically make four to five attempts per year).[8] Let's slow down, take a deep breath, choose a plan that makes sense, and then learn to follow through on it.

WHAT I DID
THAT WAS UNIQUE

HERE'S WHAT MADE MY attempt at weight loss work so well:

1. I got to know myself really, really well.
2. I used that knowledge at all times, constantly preparing ahead of time to overcome my current habits and weaknesses.
3. Through preparation, I was able to interrupt my previous patterns before they occurred and then replace those patterns with healthier ones that have lasted to this day.

This may sound simple, and it is!

It all starts here: If you want to know what a person (you) will do today, the most reliable predictor of that is what that person (you) did yesterday. Yet *everyone* seems to forget this fact when they're trying to change their habits! In his New York Times bestselling book, *The Power of Habit,* author Charles Duhigg reported that more than 40 percent of the actions we perform each day are the product not of deliberate decisions but of habit, and many of these rote activities work against what we consciously desire, as when we put too much food on our plate despite wanting to lose weight.[9] Moreover, numerous psychology studies have shown that "past behavior is the best predictor of future behavior."[10]

Let's look at it a different way. Did you ever see a werewolf movie and notice that after the wolf transforms back to a human, his clothes are all ripped up? You'd think that after the first ripped-up set of clothes, this guy would catch on and think, *Hmmm…I'm a werewolf, so I'd better get used to that. When there's a full moon, I'm going to ditch the outfit so I don't rip up so many shirts.* As much as we have an envious hate for that guy in the *Twilight* movies who's all attractive and muscly and never seems to have a shirt, you have to hand it to him – he's pretty smart. He *knows he's a werewolf,* so he leaves that shirt off before it gets all ripped up. He's a lot smarter than the Incredible Hulk, who always seems to rip through his clothes.

You and I have a tendency to live our lives like the first werewolf, with the ripped-up clothes:

We know what we're likely to do, yet when we decide to improve our weight (or finances, or anything), we blindly assume our habits will just change because we want them to. That is stupid.

To quote Susan Scott's book, *Fierce Conversations,* "What are you pretending not to know?"[11]

Pretending *not* to know things that you actually do know is stupid.

We *know* we are going to get hungry and search the cabinets and the refrigerator for sugary foods, so why do we stay stocked-up on treats? We *know* we're going to get hungry at lunch and eat fast food, so why don't we prepare a healthy lunch we'll look forward to, instead of just thinking we'll change overnight and start craving vegetables? (I can't tell you how many times someone has said, "That smells good," as I warm up a very healthy lunch that they could have easily prepared, while they pass by with unhealthy vending machine food!) We'll prepare or buy some super-healthy yet awful-tasting smoothie that we *pretend* we're going to eat, and when it's time for lunch and our coworkers are headed out, we head out the door with the green drink still in the fridge (admit it, you've done this in some form).

The point is, we pretend we *don't* know what we're going to do, and we end up underprepared when the time comes to make good choices. This isn't surprising – research published in *Annals of Behavioral Medicine* actually shows that we will avoid learning new information if it will create an obligation to do something unpleasant.[12] In short, not only do we pretend to not know what we know about ourselves, but we're compelled to not think about it too much, because it could cause us to need to make some unpleasant changes!

The good news is, there are techniques we can employ to overcome this!

MEET DERRICK,
MY ALTER EGO

LET'S HAVE SOME FUN with this. Pay attention here, because this theme is going to carry through the entire book.

My name is Eric.

I also sometimes transform into my own evil twin – a twin who drinks beer, eats pizza, watches movies, doesn't exercise, and goes to bed with a very full stomach. Let's say that "evil twin" or "werewolf" or "alter-ego" version of me will be "Derrick."

There is a version of "me" I always want to be, who is disciplined, who exercises, who writes books, and who makes healthy choices. I'm going to allow myself to call that version "Eric," because that's the guy who I hope Eric can someday always live as.

If you're a Superman fan, picture Derrick as the version that gets around red Kryptonite and starts beating up good guys. If you're a fan of Muppets Most Wanted, picture Derrick as Kermit's evil twin. I'd like for Derrick to go away, and I've spent a lot of time figuring out how to make that happen on a daily basis.

Are you with me?

Let's go back and apply the Eric/Derrick model to a scenario I already gave you.

Eric will wake up in the morning and use his Vitamix blender to prepare a healthy juice blend full of vitamins, minerals, plants, and seeds. Eric knows this juice will taste disgusting, but it's good for him, so he prepares it anyway. Eric probably read some article in *Men's Health* describing why all the things that just went into that fancy blender will make him stronger, faster, and richer.[13] Eric, at 7:00 A.M., can't wait to drink this smoothie for lunch because he knows it will be nutritious and he thinks it will give him abs. Here's the problem:

Eric doesn't eat lunch. Derrick eats lunch. Eric forgets that he is not making that nasty shake for Eric. He's making it for Derrick.

Eric should *damn* well know by this point in his life that Derrick isn't going to drink that smoothie. Derrick is going to laugh about the smoothie, leave it in the refrigerator, and either not eat anything at all or run to the vending area and grab something filling and entirely unhealthy. If we're lucky, Derrick might even feel guilty about not drinking that shake, but Derrick is certainly not going to ingest the thing. If Derrick does not have appetizing food in front of him the moment he gets hungry, he'll get absorbed in his work, skip lunch, and wait until 5:00 P.M., at which point he will go to happy hour and scarf down appetizers. Eric still exists at this point, but he's more along for the ride than anything. Both guys are hungry, and Derrick can be very convincing when unfed all day.

When Eric makes a healthy shake for lunch, he is pretending *not* to know that Derrick exists. This is stupid.

The reason that we often fail at weight loss (and many life changes that require significant alterations to our destructive patterns) is that we completely neglect the fact that we are in different states at different times of the day, and we fail to prepare for that. A large and growing body of research including studies published in *Psychology of Addictive Behaviors* and *Personality and Psychology Review* suggests that self-control is a limited resource that can be "depleted" by previous use.[14] More simply put, when you make one good, healthy decision in the morning, it may be harder to make another good, healthy decision later in the day! We know we're going to be undisciplined, so let's be ready for it.

The great Sun Tzu advised, "If you know [the enemy] and know yourself, you will not be imperiled in a hundred battles… If you do not know [the enemy] and do not know yourself, you will be imperiled in every single battle."[15] If you were in competition with an opponent, you'd want to know everything about him or her, right?

Well, in this case, you actually *are* facing an opponent (your unhealthy habits) and you actually *do* know everything about that person! *Everything!*

**You are your own worst enemy, and you
just happen to know this enemy, quite literally,
"inside and out."**

You know your opponent's every habit, every breath,
and every move. You know what he or she dreams about.
You even know how he or she will feel and react given most
situations that arise on any given day.

Pretending that we'll act differently tomorrow than
we did today for some magical reason is *absurd*, yet it's a
mistake that we all make when we attempt to change our
habits!

**The good news is that we are able to harness the
information we have about ourselves and use it to
our advantage!**

We have already determined that we are very likely to
do today what we did yesterday. That may initially make
you feel powerless, but it's the quite the opposite. Knowing
this is extremely powerful.

Have you met you? It's time to.

Now, what can we do with this information?

USING KNOWLEDGE
TO OUR ADVANTAGE

LOOK AT YOU RIGHT now – sitting there all studious, reading a book on weight loss! You're being such a mature and productive human being! It's probably hard to imagine that in a few hours you could be devouring a sleeve of bagels, Forrest-Gumping a box of chocolates, or plowing through three glasses of scotch and a quart of beef lo mein. But if we're being honest today, book or no book, that's probably what you're headed for later.

If you're anything like me, there are some self-destructive behaviors that have been limiting you for years – if not for your whole life – that you just can't seem to ditch. You and I can talk rationally while you're sitting here in your chair, with your good posture and your Brita bottle, but things won't be so rational when you're starving and it's 10:00 P.M. and there's a gallon of ice cream nine feet away.

Every day, for years, we've repeated the same behaviors. We've, at times, believed that just because we started reading a book, we would do something differently. We've allowed ourselves to believe that sheer willpower would carry us through, but the reality we've encountered is that it won't.

We need to rely on something more powerful to change our habits, and that power comes from knowledge and preparation. We will use that knowledge of exactly what you'll do in three hours to your advantage.

Instead of assuming we will change, let's flip this scenario on its head and assume that we will *not* change! Instead, let's find ways to "trick" our alter egos into doing the right things!

Let's start with an easy practice that I use on a regular basis to overcome Derrick's perpetual pizza binges.

I know Derrick loves pizza. If Derrick is hungry anywhere in the vicinity of 8:00 to 10:00 P.M., Derrick will use our laptop to get online and order a pizza on our credit card. (Derrick is like the worst roommate in the world, but we share a body instead of a room.) When this time of the evening rolls around, if Eric hasn't taken steps to have something ready for Derrick to eat that makes him not think of pizza anymore, both of us are going to gain a pound or more overnight.

So here's what Eric learned to do:

Eric started to experiment and found that if he could eat enough healthy food at 4:00, while he's still "himself" at the office, Derrick isn't even feeling very hungry until 9:00. As long as Eric can get to bed before 9:00 or leave Derrick a healthy snack that he'll opt for over pizza, the two of us will be golden. This works most of the time – but not all the time.

Just in case Derrick still wants that pizza, Eric has a backup plan. Eric knows that if he can spend some time in the early morning hours or even on the weekend making his own frozen pizzas using whole wheat tortillas for crust, piling veggies (including green olives, one of Derrick's favorite toppings) onto it, and making sure to use a tiny bit of cheese and just a spoonful of very low-sugar pizza sauce, Derrick will use that to satisfy his cravings. If Derrick gets hungry enough to eat, and the snack isn't enough, he'll go for one of these frozen pizzas because they're faster than the delivery guy. If that happens, we've won. We don't gain the pounds and, at worst, we maintain our weight overnight.

A quick note of caution just for HCG protocol followers: do not eat the little pizzas on Phase 2 of the HCG plan, thinking they're okay. Check with your nutritionist first. For me, these cause a "plateau" effect, where my weight was maintained. That's just fine when you're trying to maintain your weight, but it's not good in Phase 2 when you're trying to drop weight quickly. I'll get into more detail on this later.

The mistake many of us make – and that I've made many times in my life – is to sit here, in our productive, weight loss-book-reading, mature states, thinking that we'll be in the same state in five hours and not preparing for it. We say to ourselves, I just have to stop eating pizzas at night, then I'll lose weight, but we do nothing to prepare ourselves to replace the behavior or make the change! This is just one example and there are many more to discuss.

The key to success in weight loss – or in any habit-change – is to find ways of changing our habits that actually work, instead of just trying to harness some form of willpower that we want to just magically appear. Instead of focusing on things that seem like they'll work, let's do things that just work.

Here's an example to illustrate what works, and what doesn't work. Do you have one of those "dingers" in your car that rings like crazy when you aren't wearing a seatbelt? These dingers are one of the most annoying things in the world, but I'll tell you what – they certainly make me put my seatbelt on!

Remember back in the '80s and '90s (if you're old enough to follow me here) how there used to be commercials showing people who had been severely injured or died from not wearing a seatbelt? How about the billboards by the highway that read, "Click it or ticket"? It's cute. It rhymes. Whoever thought that up was probably very clever, thinking, *If people would just remember they're supposed to do this, they'll do it.* The problem is, I could watch those commercials and see the billboards all day, but as soon as I was in the car wearing a shirt that was about to get wrinkled by a seatbelt, I was not about to "click it." As much as those ideas sounded like they would work, they didn't work (on me). For me, it was the *dinger* that worked. For me, it was an annoying, constantly-ringing, never-ending bell sound that made me do something that would save my life. It's funny, I know. You would think that the threat of massive consequences would make me change my behavior. The *truth* is that it doesn't. The threat of a heart attack doesn't stop us from eating burgers. The threat of obesity doesn't stop us from drinking soda all day at work. We don't need solutions that *should* work! Instead, we need more dingers. We need to *create* dingers in every area of our lives, to keep us on track.

In order to change behavior, we need to get a little creative and find a better way. We need solutions that work like the dinger.

What works for you when it comes to crushing your bad habits? It's for you to figure out. You need to experiment like crazy, think, get creative, and do what it takes. Realizing that you'll need to do this brings you a giant step closer to losing weight than you were when you thought you "just needed to change."

This is going to take planning. We know our enemy, we plan, and we prepare for that enemy to arrive! When Bruce Banner (you) turns into the Incredible Hulk (whatever your name for your Derrick is), we know exactly how green he gets, where he tends to wander, and what he tends to beat up. Better, we know exactly how to deal with that situation because we see it coming.

In short, preparation becomes our key to change.

Using preparation to our advantage, we can turn the tables! The Boy Scout Motto, *Be Prepared*, is the basis for our whole discussion. With proper preparation, we can win the battle with our werewolf, with the Incredible Hulk, with Derrick, or with whomever it is that is your alter ego.

Let's look at some more examples.

Example: Rising Early

Eric knows that when it comes to eating, he turns into Derrick every night at 9:00. Eric, on purpose, will get up extremely early in the morning, so that he gets sleepy by 8:00 and is lights-out in bed long before Derrick arrives.

Example: Sunday Brunch

Let's apply this to you. You've been invited to brunch on Sunday morning. You love the restaurant your friends are going to because they have great desserts. Here's the easiest way to turn a potential disaster into a healthy Sunday morning: **don't go.** You can make all the excuses in the world about staying close to your friends and not wanting to go to the extreme, but if you can't sacrifice a brunch in a four-week period of weight loss, then you're not ready to start this in the first place. In this scenario, you need to know yourself well enough to realize that if you show up at that brunch, the dessert is as good as in your belly. I'll mention at this point that this is temporary. You can happily go to brunch again with your friends, once you've lost the weight you want to lose and are comfortable in your maintenance phase.

> **Don't set yourself up to rely on willpower.**
> **Don't pretend you don't know you.**

Example: Happy Hour

Eric knows that, after work, there are two coworkers who will always come up with a reason to go out for appetizers and drinks, to talk about something work-related. He also knows that Derrick will always agree to go along with them and that it's impossible for Derrick to say no when they ask him to join. So, during the weight loss phase, what did Eric do? He left the office before those guys, every single day, and would shut his phone off until he was safely at home, so that Derrick couldn't answer it. Yes, Eric missed his friends, and yes, it wasn't polite, but it worked, and Eric realized he had to do it in order to create change.

Example: Leaving Before the Stress

Similar to the story above – and as we've discussed – Eric knows that if he has an early, healthy dinner while still at work and leaves work at about 4:45 P.M. following a nine- or ten-hour day, he'll go home and get some rest. Eric knows that if he stays at work until 7:00, Derrick is going to believe he deserves a cocktail, and he's going to head out with the guys. A Derrick who has been at work for 12 hours will *undoubtedly* talk himself into heading out to dinner instead of going home for something healthy. Because of this, Eric is very, very careful to leave work at a reasonable hour unless there's a very good reason not to.

Example: Exercise

As you might guess by now, Derrick also hates exercise and refuses to do it. Sometimes (and I bet you can relate to this one), Eric will lay out his running shoes and a whole running outfit in the shape of a little Eric-made-of-clothes on the floor, then set his alarm clock for 4:00 A.M., so that he can get up and get a nice run in. It's Derrick who hears the alarm at 4:00, and who then curses or laughs at Eric, and proceeds through a hazy 15 pushes of the snooze button. Derrick is not getting out of bed, and he's certainly not putting on his running shoes. Here's the trick Eric used for that. Eric put a small energy drink next to the bed and woke up at 3:30 A.M. Derrick may not put on running shoes or shorts, but he's aware enough to drink an energy drink early in the morning. When the drink hits the bloodstream, it opens Eric's eyes (which would have been Derrick's eyes) about 30 minutes later, and the two of us charge out into the dark for a run. I do not recommend this method to you because it is probably not healthy – definitely check with your doctor before thinking about using energy drinks regularly. In fact, a number of adverse events relating to energy drink use, including some deaths allegedly caused by energy drinks, have been reported to the FDA.[16] This was just one trick that Eric used to keep Derrick at bay, and I felt it was worth including for you. Later in the book I'll explain a healthier way to get yourself moving in the morning, which pretty much consists of changing your body clock in such a way that you're naturally rising earlier over time. On a positive side note, I actually was able to stop drinking energy drinks altogether during this program, by drinking more sparkling water as a replacement!

Example: Movie Money

Here's an example that's outside of the weight loss realm. Eric knows that if he's bored and has nothing to do at night, Derrick will rent an on-demand movie, and these movies typically are overpriced. As you've learned, Derrick can be an impulsive jerk – an impulsive jerk who happens to love movies. To solve this, Eric bought Derrick a Netflix subscription, through which movies are delivered on a regular basis through the mail. It's a monthly expense, but it's far less than Derrick's on-demand movies. As long as Eric stays on top of the queue and makes sure good movies are always in line to be delivered next, Derrick always has something to watch without breaking the budget.

Example: Using Strong Hours

Eric knows that from early morning until about 11:00 A.M. daily, he's insanely productive. After that, Derrick takes over and starts procrastinating and doing almost nothing. Eric uses this to his advantage. Eric never plans to do a hard task or a challenging meeting at 3:00 P.M., because he knows it will be on Derrick to get that task done or to attend that meeting, and Derrick is terrible at that sort of thing. Derrick is excellent at tiny, menial tasks that need to get done but don't require much thought or effort. For that reason, Eric assigns all of his menial, thoughtless tasks to times of the day when Derrick is around. Writing a manuscript? That's Eric's work. Checking email and responding with single sentences? That's Derrick, all afternoon.

Example: Homework and Laundry

Here's another one. Eric knows that when has homework or writing to do, Derrick will end that idea, real fast, if he's in a place where there are distractions. Eric will sit down at the computer at home to start his homework, and sometimes within seconds Derrick will appear. Derrick will rise from that same computer and walk over to start doing laundry, clean the house, rearrange groceries, or worse – make himself a drink. You'll know Eric has homework due when Derrick has cleaned the entire house, has folded all the laundry, and is drinking wine on the couch, watching a whole TV series on Netflix. Now, Eric knows that when he drives himself to a Starbucks, Barnes and Noble, or Whole Foods and sits down with some coffee or maybe even a glass of cabernet, there is almost nothing for Derrick to do at any of those places. Derrick might try to browse the Internet or talk to other customers, but he's not really that bad when he's out in public. This gives Eric plenty of time, without distraction, to finish his homework assignments. He'll give

Derrick a coffee to keep him calm, and he'll bust through a paper. Knowing this fact, Eric is very careful to get himself to a place where Derrick won't come out, before he starts his homework. Doing anything else would be idiotic and evidence of Eric pretending not to know himself at all.

Your Turn

As much fun as it just may have been for you to get a glimpse into my quirky life, we both know you have an alter-ego as well. Is your name Kelly, and do you have a Shelly to assign some things to? Is your name Gary, and do you have a Jerry in your mind who loves eating pies? Whoever it is and whoever you are, get to know yourself and do some thinking on this. When you focus on it, get intentional about changing, and really think through solutions, it can be fun!

Give it some thought! When that craving hits so hard that we forget all of our goals and aspirations and we just want to eat that treat in front of us, order that pizza, or refuse to head to the gym, what are we going to do? No longer will we rely on thinking we'll just choose differently in the face of temptation. Let's prepare! What are you *really, really going to do?* What's your replacement behavior? What tools are you going to arm yourself with ahead of time?

Some of these suggestions may work for you, and some may not. Whatever the case may be, it's up to you to know yourself, get creative, and think of ways to stop your nasty alter ego from ruining your life, *way* before it's time to face the temptation. It's about staying ahead of yourself! I can't give you specifics that will work for every scenario, but I'm 100 percent positive that *you* know yourself well enough that you can take some time to make a plan and give yourself those specifics. The rest of this book will be about how I made this work in my life and can serve as a guide that you can adapt to your own life.

IT'S NOT AS BAD AS IT SOUNDS

WITH ALL THIS TALK about how difficult it is to change who we are, it's not hopeless. Changing who we are *is* possible – we're not *actually* werewolves. In fact, research in the *International Journal of Obesity* shows that a behavioral weight loss intervention monitored by physicians can result in significant weight loss as well as improvements in the ability to restrain eating, and increase activity![17] Research also shows that there is a strong correlation between significant weight loss and craving reductions of foods. The body is actually craving less and less harmful, fatty foods as it is losing weight, helping itself lose even more weight and adjust to a new lifestyle.[18]

In other words, when you persist and lose the weight, it gets easier to control your inner wolf.

I didn't write the advice in the "werewolf/Eric/Derrick" format to discourage you, but instead, I wrote it because I believe knowing ourselves is the first step of transformation.

As people, I believe we can change and then develop new habits. Let's not be tricked into assuming those habits will just change overnight, because they don't! Let's admit how difficult it is to overcome temptation on sheer will-power. Let's use that knowledge to our advantage. Let's get creative. Let's use logic. Let's use preparedness. Let's use every tool we have in the toolbox up here in our heads and dominate our alter egos so that they have no choice but to come along for the ride, and then ride that wave of change to permanent transformation that can be carried through life.

Let's know that we'll be weak and trust first that the weakness will come, but also know in the back of our minds that we'll be prepared to overcome our weakness with our passion, our creativity, and our planning.

By the end of my transformation, Derrick wasn't around nearly as often as he was at the beginning. Because I found creative ways to keep Derrick at bay for an extended period of time, I found that he just didn't come around as much anymore. I hope that this advice can do the same for you.

By the way, even though he's not around all the time, Derrick still lurks a bit. I'll admit that as I originally typed these words, I paused for 20 minutes to run and pick up some M&M's, even though I didn't want any. That's because I knew that Derrick has recently learned that the frozen yogurt shop reopened across the street, and if there were M&M's around later tonight, he would eat those instead of walking over there. M&M's may not be nutritious, but if they keep Derrick away from that frozen yogurt shop, it's a win.

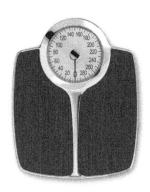

PART 2:
ABOUT HCG

BEFORE WE GET INTO any more details, I'd like to first give you some background about what HCG is, what phases the program consists of, and some of the benefits of the program. We'll discuss the massive benefit of the highly prescriptive nature of the program, as well as exercise and overall health aspects.

HCG: THE THEORY, CONTROVERSY, AND LACK OF ANY DECENT EVIDENCE

ACCORDING TO HCGDIETCOUNCIL.ORG, DR. ATW Simeons discovered the potential benefits of Human Chorionic Gonadotropin, or HCG, when he began to observe women in third-world countries. He observed that even though the women were working in fields and malnourished, their babies were still born healthy and at full weight. Dr. Simeons attributed this to the hormone HCG. Simeons began to use HCG to treat boys with low testosterone levels. Simeons observed that the boys slimmed down and lost fat, specifically in the abdomen. Dr. S. went on to find that both men and women could lose fat in short periods of time by using HCG in combination with a very low calorie diet.[19] Dr. Simeons went on to publish the book, *Pounds and Inches, A New Approach to Obesity*, where he recommended a system of pairing the administration of HCG with a low carbohydrate, low calorie diet to facilitate weight loss.[20]

Fast forward to now. HCG seems to be the growing trend in weight loss these days, as more people are getting the injectable HCG prescribed for them. It's become so popular that Dr. Oz even did a number of video vignettes with HCG as a focus.[21] HCG is being sold on the market in multiple forms. It can be taken orally, or through injections. "HCG droplets" which are administered under the tongue, seem to be popular. A lot of websites and experts will tell you that the injected HCG is the only type to use because it's the most potent and it actually is HCG. Others favor drops that are placed under the tongue. There are some over-the-counter products that contain no HCG, but make claims about producing HCG in your system. Again, to be clear, I can't recommend any of these to you because I'm not a doctor, and I think you should consult with a nutritionist before moving ahead with any form of this plan.

Now, it's no secret that HCG is controversial. Some people claim to have had success with it. A 1995 study published in the *British Journal of Clinical Pharmacology* showed that HCG only had a placebo effect.[22] This means that patients using a substitute for HCG had the same result as those to whom real HCG was administered. In other words, if you injected yourself with saline or, to be arbitrary, chanted a mantra of your choice three times a day, while following the other instructions of the HCG diet plan, you'd have the same results.

As Dr. Zach LaBoube explains in *Don't Starve, Eat Smart, and Lose: A Modern Adaptation of the HCG Diet*, the most common misunderstanding is that the HCG, in and of itself, produces weight loss, which is untrue. The weight loss is actually a result of decreased caloric intake, and the role of the HCG is targeted weight loss wherein muscle mass is maintained while unwanted fat is dropped. Also according to Dr. Zach, the HCG facilitates an entirely healthy metabolic process called ketosis, and although this is facilitated by HCG, optimal levels can only be achieved by limiting carbohydrates (which is done as part of the HCG protocol).[23]

Here's what I have to say about it:

For me, losing 29.1 pounds in 38 days happened.[24] In my own clinical test, using an insanely invalid sample size of 1 (yet valid for me), the HCG diet was 100 percent effective.

Now, any logical person will tell you that correlation does not imply causation. Just because something happened while something else happened doesn't mean one thing was because of the other. You can drink a gallon of milk on the same day your neighbor lets you borrow his Chrysler Sebring, but that does not mean that if you drink a gallon of milk tomorrow, your neighbor will again offer you his whip. These two things probably have nothing to do with each other. I mean, they could, but you have no evidence to show that they do.

During my weight loss period, I injected myself with HCG every morning. At the same time, I was taking in somewhere between 500 and 800 calories per day, as prescribed by my nutritionist (it's worth noting here that this was supervised and required weekly check-ins). So, is it possible that the caloric deficit could have had the same result without the HCG injections? It's quite possible, but I can't say for certain. What I *do* know is that for whatever reason, the collective set of actions I took throughout the 38-day period did cause me to lose the weight.

Being very honest, if I were to attempt to lose more weight at this point, I would use all of the techniques

I've included in this book, using a diet prescribed by my nutritionist, without the HCG. Why? Having now spent a lot of time learning about the ways that specific foods and changes to my daily caloric intake affect my weight, I would tell you that for me, the nutritional counseling I received, combined with the approaches to habit-changing that I developed, seemed to be the "active ingredient" in my comprehensive plan. I do believe that the initial period of weight loss *may* have been affected by the HCG hormone, but I'm also now confident that I am personally capable of using the techniques described in this book to lose weight without the HCG hormone. The question remains, could I have learned all of this and experienced the initial weight loss without the HCG? I cannot answer that.

Therefore, I think it's worth it for you to discuss this decision with your doctor and nutritionist to decide what will work best for you. The point of my writing this book is not to convince you to use or not to use HCG, but instead, to show you that my rapid weight loss sparked habit changes that have persisted, and ultimately changed my life.

Important reminder: I can't recommend this for you because I'm not a doctor, and only a doctor can prescribe the injectable stuff I used.

THE RISKS OF HCG

IT'S IMPORTANT THAT BEFORE beginning any diet plan, including the HCG diet, you discuss the risks with your doctor and nutritionist. Before I started on this plan, I conducted research to determine whether or not this was even a good idea.

One website pointed out that side effects might include headaches, depression, restlessness, increased risk of blood clots, and also some symptoms of pregnancy, including water retention and swelling and sensitive breasts.[25] Another site reported that restlessness might occur, as well as leg cramps, constipation, and temporary hair thinning.[26] Medical research cited in *Seminars In Reproductive Medicine* also showed that there is a potential risk for women called OHSS, or ovarian hyperstimulation syndrome, in which ovaries over-stimulated by hormones could swell and leak fluid into the abdomen.[27]

The other risks I discovered tended to have to do with an ultra-low-calorie diet more than they had to do with the HCG hormone itself. Specifically, there were reports of fainting, and even one report to the FDA of someone who had developed a pulmonary embolism (a blood clot in the lung that can be fatal). Other side effects of such a low-calorie diet can range from bone and muscle loss to imbalances in electrolytes to gallstones to death.[28]

The more prominent worries that critics seem to have is that there are products out there that are sold under the HCG name but are not really HCG, and that people using the HCG diet will gain the weight back.

Of all of these risks, the one I would like to speak to is the risk of gaining the weight back. I'm certain that it exists, and that's one of the reasons I've written this book. Because of the techniques I employed, and because of the great accountability provided to me by my healthcare team, I didn't gain the weight back, while I changed habits in my life that are certain to keep me on the right course. I now cook healthy foods, and my nutritional habits are entirely different than they were prior to starting this diet. Though gaining the weight back is a risk, I think you and I have the chance to prove a lot of doubters wrong by maintaining our progress.

The reason I bring up these risks is because I want to give you a starting point to do your own research and decide, in collaboration with your doctor and nutritionist, if this type of plan is right for you. I can't make that decision for you. I made the decision for myself, and I personally did not experience most of these side effects, with the exception of some hunger and moodiness, which I'll cover later in the book.

A GENERAL OVERVIEW OF THE PLAN I FOLLOWED

THOUGH I WON'T OFFER you the details of my plan, because I require that you get those from another book or medical professional, I will give you the basics, in layman's terms, so you can follow along.

Phase 1

In Phase 1, which covered the first two days of my plan, I ate a ton of food. This was the "binge" phase, in which I gorged myself with food in order to (according to my nutritionist) build up some fat stores and to prepare to not be so hungry in the first week of Phase 2. The HCG injections started on Day 1 of Phase 1. The injections are a lot easier than I thought they would be. After one or two, I was completely used to it. The needle is tiny, and it really doesn't hurt. Conversely, it makes you feel kind of like Ivan Drago in *Rocky IV*. I think a lot of people freak out about the injections and feel like that just isn't an option. To me, the injections helped me to stay focused. After injecting myself with a hormone in the morning, I was much more likely to rethink cheating on my diet plan in the afternoon!

Phase 2

Phase 2 is the low-calorie, weight loss phase of the HCG Diet plan. In Phase 2, I would eat about 500 to 800 calories per day, touching almost no starches (breads, potatoes, etc.) and drinking almost no alcohol (we'll talk about my cheating later). This lasted for about 38 days, and this is the period during which I actually lost the weight. The HCG injections continued from Phase 1, were performed daily during Phase 2, and ended at the end of Phase 2. I did not exercise at all during Phase 2.

Phase 3

Phase 3 is the "transition phase," where I stopped injecting myself with HCG and increased my caloric intake to about 1,800 calories per day. This lasted for about three weeks. During Phase 3, I continued to avoid starches, as I had in Phase 2. The difference was that I ate a lot *more* of the healthy foods I had gotten used to in Phase 2. I also was able to add in oils and nuts that I hadn't eaten in Phase 2. In Phase 3, I did begin to drink a little alcohol again, but as you'll read later, my tastes had changed dramatically, and I rarely drank beer or hard liquor, substituting in red wine instead. I did exercise during Phase 3 and actually completed a half-marathon during this time period.

Phase 4

Phase 4 was referred to by my nutritionist as "the rest of your life." I'm therefore, by definition, still in Phase 4. In this phase, I maintained my new tastes and eating habits while adding in all sorts of new foods, from starches to dairy to fruits and vegetables. I created menus with a great deal of variety. I continue to this day to "test" how my body handles different foods and to make changes to include foods I love while maintaining a healthier weight and higher energy levels. In Phase 4, nothing is off-limits anymore, and the calorie restriction is entirely gone. It's more about monitoring your own reactions to foods and knowing yourself well enough to make adjustments when needed. I've now lost even more weight while in Phase 4, just by closely watching what I eat during periods when I want to trim down a bit.

THE GREAT THING ABOUT HCG'S HIGHLY PRESCRIPTIVE NATURE

IN ORDER FOR THE HCG plan to work for me, I had to learn to trust the system, blindly, with absolute faith. That's all part of it. I look at the prescriptive nature of this plan as a benefit! Think about it: a doctor or nutritionist *is* going to tell you *exactly* what to do, and if you do it, it's going to work. It's that simple. The downside of this is that you need to give yourself over to something that just won't feel right at times.

When you hit Phase 2 and you're not eating much at all, you'll be thinking *there's no way this can be right*, and you might start to question what's happening. Don't do that.

Also, when you hit Phase 3 and you need to start upping your calories like crazy, you (again) might be thinking, *There's no way this can be right.* You might (yet again) start to question what's happening. You may be tempted to continue to keep your calories low because you're scared of gaining the weight back. Again, don't do that.

I'll say it again for emphasis.

**You need to learn to trust the system,
blindly, with absolute faith.**

It goes further. You need to find a team of healthcare professionals you trust, including a doctor and a nutrition-ist. Then, you need to do exactly what your nutritionist tells you, even if it initially seems strange to you. Remember, we became overweight from our bad habits. If something isn't "normal" to you, that just may be a good thing! If your nutritionist tells you to eat lima beans, you eat them. You eat exactly what she tells you to. If you're full of lima beans and you can't eat another bite, but she told you to eat a certain number of bites, you eat another bite. If something bothers you about what has been prescribed, then you stick to the advice until you're able to discuss other options or substitutes with your nutritionist. You don't make up some rationale in your head for why you need to deviate for now. You don't deviate for now.

I believe that this principle is why this plan worked so well for me. This plan is insanely prescriptive. I needed that. I needed someone to tell me exactly what to do, and she did, and I did it, and it worked. In order for it to work, I needed to have absolute blind faith. Once I let it work for me, I began to love it.

One thing you may be tempted to do is to try to inject your own knowledge into your interpretation of this plan.

You may also be tempted to listen to advice from people who are not your doctor or nutritionist. You may read something in a magazine or a book that sounds right, but it's not a part of the plan. Don't do it. Stay the course. **Stay the course.** *Stay the course.*

You'll be tempted to deviate! You may even convince yourself that you're doing something unhealthy. Think about the massive mix of "health" advice out there! We've heard it all by now: "Calorie counting matters." "Calorie counting doesn't matter." "Eat healthy fats." "Don't eat too much fat." "Lift weights, running breaks down muscle." "Running builds muscle." "Carbo load." "Don't eat carbohydrates." "Do interval training instead of distance running." "Run a marathon." "Eat three meals a day." "Eat six meals a day." "Don't snack between meals." "Have a healthy snack between meals to curb hunger." "Extra calories add up." "Good calories make you feel full." "Be vegan." "Vegans need more iron." "Animal protein is needed." "Animal protein causes cancer." "The dinosaurs died because of animal protein." The list is unending.

There is so much research out there in the world that, to me, it seems impossible to navigate the path toward good health without the help of experts. Even experts constantly disagree with one another!

What you need is a highly prescriptive, holistic plan that overarches your entire way of living, eating, and being.

What advice do you follow? I will tell you what advice to follow. You follow the advice of your doctor and nutritionist. These are professionals who spend their lives interpreting the research and working with real people who trust them to get real results.

The best part of this advice is that there's no longer any confusion. You've given yourself over to a plan that you can trust will work, and therefore, you have a good reason to overcome all of the nagging questions in your mind. You've heard again and again that eating breakfast is important to weight loss, but sometimes you're standing there in the morning thinking, *I'm not hungry now, so should I really be eating a lot of food?* You now know that if your nutritionist told you to eat a lot of food, you should do it, and you can trust that it will work! The little voices in your head can now rest, and you can silence them, all the while knowing that you'll get the results you want. There's no more guess and check. There's no more experimentation. You've found something you know will work. Now it's time to trust it and move forward with confidence!

Another great part about this strategy is that a good nutritionist won't cave to the societal norms, and for that reason, she may tell you to do (or not to do) some things that may sound strange or even extreme. I'll give you an example. When I first went to visit my nutritionist and she laid out the meal plan, I immediately asked if I could have lunch meat, like turkey or chicken from the deli.

"Why do you need that?" she asked.

"Don't eat it," my nutritionist told me. Then she pointed me back to the paper in my hand, outlining the plan.

The research points to my nutritionist being right-on here. I later read that heavily processed foods contain synthetic chemicals like dyes, preservatives, and artificial flavors. The list of these chemicals currently on super-market shelves is long, while the research on their health effects is limited. We know that some people have allergic responses to individual compounds, but more serious health effects have been suggested, including risks of ADHD development.[29] Evidently, even healthy lunch meat has some chemicals in it that I just didn't need.

I then asked about bananas.

"Stay away from those," she told me. Then she suggested other fruits with less sugar in them.

As crazy as this sounds, my nutritionist even advised me to stay away from carrots, because they were somewhat high in sugar. She did mention that she'd never seen anyone get fat from eating carrots, but that it probably was best to avoid them while in Phase 2.

I'm not sure what your doctor and nutritionist will tell you to eat, but if it was anything like the advice I got, then it's advice your friends and family will question. Put it this way: I just had a nutrition professional tell me to avoid lean lunch meats like deli turkey, to stay away from carrots, and not to eat bananas during certain phases of this plan! To most people, including those people you interact with on a day-to-day basis, that advice won't sound right, and those people may try to convince you to deviate from the plan. Don't let them convince you! They're just going off of what they know, but it's not necessarily good advice for you, and that's why you've hired a professional.

I'm not saying carrots and bananas are bad foods. They're actually a healthy alternative to many of the snacks people choose regularly. My point is that the changes you need to make in order to lose weight may seem very strange to you and others around you at first. Get used to the weirdness. The plan is highly prescriptive, and your job is to follow it, not sneak around it.

Again, the whole point here is that whatever your doctor and nutritionist tell you to do, you should do, and you're going to need to get used to that fact. If you're not ready to listen to these professionals, there is not a book (and that includes this one) that will help you. When you accumulate the levels of frustration with your body that are needed to create significant changes in your life, you will have no trouble developing a willingness to follow the advice of these professionals.

COOKING: IT AIN'T SO BAD

YOU PROBABLY SAW THIS coming when you read about the ban on lunch meat. My nutritionist told me that I needed to start cooking. There was no shortcutting it. With the plan that was prescribed for me, the meats that were allowed are the kind you buy at the store and bring home and cook. My options to get this meat into a cooked state were to hire a chef to cook it or to cook it myself.

In the past, I always made excuses in my head about this. When people told me that I needed to cook, I always thought, *They don't understand my life.* I thought, *They don't get that I work 60 or more hours a week sometimes, and that I can't fit cooking in like a "normal person" can.* First, I was arrogant to think that way, because all people have busy lives, regardless of whether they're filling them with work, family, or any other obligations that are important to them. We all have priorities. Second, I was just wrong. I had *time* to cook, but I didn't previously see it as a high enough priority that I would change my other activities to do it.

Before, when someone told me that I needed to cook in order to be healthy, I would immediately dismiss the advice and start to think of workarounds. I'd try to think of ways I could get cooked food without cooking. That's not the way to be thinking if you want to have a successful transformation.

This was the most massive turnaround I had ever made in my health, and I believe it was because I began to spend time preparing food. Research backs this conclusion. Researchers in *Harvard Women's Health Watch* published commentary suggesting that the best way to keep the weight you have lost off is to consistently cook at home![30]

At this point, I realized that what I had tried before wasn't going to work anymore and that in order to make things work, I was going to need to do what my nutritionist said. She told me I needed to cook. So I went out and bought the Frigidaire version of the George Foreman grill, and I started to cook on it.

First, I tried chicken. I'd buy raw, pre-trimmed chicken from my local grocery and, every morning, I'd throw a couple of pieces on the grill, along with some asparagus. I'd put a ton of black pepper on it and no salt. This actually tasted pretty good! I tried various other seasonings as well, but I went very light on them because I didn't want to hurt my progress by over-salting anything.

After time, I started to branch out and even put some Mahi Mahi on that grill. That was great, too, and I couldn't believe it because I've never been a "fish guy." I found that after eating nothing but chicken for a few weeks, one quickly becomes a "fish guy." I now enjoy fish very much!

When I started to branch out into different vegetables, I first used my Vitamix blender to make a veggie smoothie to drink throughout the day. "Veggie smoothie" is actually stretching it because it was really just water and liquefied spinach. I instantly named this mixture "spinach water," and affectionately referred to it by that name. This came to a quick stop, because Derrick felt that the smoothies tasted like absolute garbage if they didn't have sugary fruits like pineapple in them. A lot of people who have gotten into great physical condition say that these smoothies are an acquired taste, it's just that I found grilled asparagus and green beans to be more appealing, and I haven't dedicated the time or energy to acquire this taste I've heard others speak of. I think it's a personal decision. If your doctor tells you to have vegetables, and vegetables are going into your mouth and then you are swallowing them, I think that earns you a pat on the back. I may never enjoy smoothies, so I've found other ways to eat the veggies.

As I started cooking more often, I'd also visit the grocery store more often. I had fun finding all sorts of good seasonings that didn't have added sugar, and I'd use them to season meats and vegetables.

I also really started to enjoy my morning cooking time. I'd get up, weigh in, have some coffee, get the grill started, and cook. That way, I wasn't distracted at work by having to find food or by being hungry. I always had exactly what I needed, nicely prepared, packaged, and ready to warm up (or even eat cold if I was in a hurry). It was actually a great lifestyle change, because I was no longer eating the terrible foods that just about everyone else seemed to be eating, *and* I was enjoying the food I prepared more than I had previously enjoyed the trash food from the office vending machines.

Once you're given a list of foods to prepare by your healthcare team, I highly suggest that you bite the bullet and begin cooking for yourself. Don't try to avoid it. Look it right in the eye, learn how to do it, and start enjoying that part. Get some kitchen tools like a vegetable chopper and a spiral slicer that turns squash into spaghetti (I'll go into more depth on these later). Buy some big pots and pans so you can cook more at one time and end up with healthy leftovers. Find some low-sugar seasonings you love that you can mix and match with all different foods. Find ways to make your cooking more flavorful while keeping it healthy! In my experience, there is no way other than this. Don't try it. Just do it.

EXERCISE, LACK THEREOF, AND FOCUS

I'VE ALREADY MENTIONED THAT I did not exercise during the 38 days I was in Phase 2 of the plan. According to my nutritionist, exercising during a time of such low calorie intake wasn't advisable, and could even cause my weight loss to plateau. Your doctor and nutritionist may give you similar advice, and if that's the case, you should follow it and plan to not exercise during Phase 2 of the HCG Diet.

Exercise was not the "active ingredient" in this plan, and it wasn't necessary for this weight loss phase. Research shows that exercise alone is not necessarily a driver of weight loss. In fact, though many people who want to lose weight believe they need to dedicate a lot of time to the gym, researchers have been finding that people who exercise don't necessarily lose weight. A study published in The British Journal of Sports Medicine reported that 58 obese people studied completed 12 weeks of supervised aerobic training without changing their diets. The group lost an average of a little more than seven pounds, and many lost barely half that.[31] I'm not trying to talk you out of exercising. I personally exercise regularly now, and I think you should exercise. I'm making the point here that though exercise may improve your overall health, weight loss, itself, may not be driven by exercise in the way many people who want to lose weight seem to think it is.

This made sense to me personally, because I had done a lot of running before starting the plan while eating a relatively healthy (yet not restrictive) diet, and I wasn't losing weight at all. We have all heard that muscle weighs more than fat, and that may have been a small part of the reason for my body's reluctance to become lighter while increasing my running mileage, yet I found that at the time I still had plenty of fat to lose, and it just wasn't going away.

Let me tell you – this lack of exercise was extremely relaxing. Actually, it wasn't just the lack of exercise that was relaxing, it was the lack of being guilty about not exercising that relaxed me! For the first time in my life, I was allowed to take some time off from exercise and not feel guilty about it!

Most importantly, taking this time away from the gym allowed me to focus my time on cooking and on intentionally changing my daily routine and habits.

It's counter-intuitive, I know. You've heard for your whole life that weight loss is about diet and exercise. Now, you have healthcare professionals telling you that you need to stay away from exercise for a bit. My advice is (surprise) to trust the plan given to you by your team of professionals. In this case, if they tell you that exercise might harm your progress because you're not taking in enough calories to sustain the level of exertion required for exercise, you need to listen. If your healthcare professionals tell you that what I'm saying is not right and that you should exercise, you need to listen! You already know the theme here. What your doctor and nutritionist say, goes.

I'll digress for just a moment to make this point – if you're using the HCG protocol, you will probably hear from your doctor and nutritionist that the stoppage of exercise is only in Phase 2. That's just a short period of time, and once you get through the weight loss period, you will most likely be instructed to start exercising again! If that's the case, do it!

If you believe this book is about being lazy and not ever exercising, while being able to lose weight, you are mistaken!

If you're using this program correctly, it's to get you a jump-start on a healthy lifestyle, where exercise is a regular part of your week!

I found that Phase 2 caused me to look *forward* to the days in Phase 3 when I would be able to both eat more and work out more! Now, exercise is again a regular part of my lifestyle, and it comes as a second priority only to getting the right healthy foods cooked and into my body.

You don't want to lose weight and end up without the muscle and endurance reserves to be able to sustain that weight loss, right? The HCG plan, in my opinion, is not a "shortcut," if used correctly. Exercise and activity are still a big part of your ultimate health, and just because you won't exercise for a bit on Phase 2, doesn't mean that you shouldn't get started again once you get to Phase 3. Look forward to vigorous activity at 30 pounds lighter!!!

There's another benefit I found to focusing less on the gym during my weight loss phase. When I spent less time worrying about fitting in my workouts, I was able to direct more of my focus on preparing the right foods, as I've mentioned, and also on *getting enough sleep!* Research published in the *American Journal of Clinical Nutrition* showed that sleep is beneficial for weight loss, and that weight loss is beneficial for sleep – talk about a powerful chain reaction to start![32]

Before, when I had tried to lose weight, I spent a lot of time and energy getting to the gym every day or running outside. This sucked up many valuable hours, and it caused me many times to eat even worse foods than I would have, and sometimes to deprive myself of an hour or two of sleep so I could get to the gym. Now, after having success with the HCG diet, I look at exercise and fitness in an entirely different way. I now separate my exercise and fitness goals from my body weight goals. I believe that even though these two areas of focus may be beneficial to each other, that *specific focus is needed in both of these areas, separately.*

Here's how I see it. If you want to lose weight, focus on losing weight. If you want to run a marathon, focus on marathon training. Focus on what you want to accomplish and don't intermix the goals unless they truly, absolutely, perfectly align.

When you take a step back and look at the different goals of marathon running and weight loss, you might realize that they do not fully align with the same sets of actions. You might actually compromise your weight loss goals by training to run a marathon. Likewise, you might compromise your marathon goals by trying to lose weight!

At times, these two things may actually pull you in different directions! Specifically, you may find that you need to increase your caloric intake to be a better marathoner, and you may retain weight by stressing your body with marathon training. As a matter of fact, when it comes to marathon training specifically, *Competitor Magazine* suggested that while in the midst of training, runners should aim at a more moderately paced weight loss of a half-pound to one pound per week, which entails a 250-500 daily calorie restriction, focused on producing moderate weight loss over time.[33]

The mistake I used to make – that I feel many people make – was mixing the two focuses. I would say to myself, *You should run a marathon so that you end up losing weight,* or, *If you train to climb another mountain, you'll lose the weight easily.* At one point in my life I was running 10 miles every day, not losing a pound, while training to summit Mt. Whitney. All along, I had not seen the conflict. I was focused on one area, trying to get results in another area. My training in the past had sometimes caused me to retain weight due to the added stress of running, as well as the added need for caloric intake.

What I needed, and what I finally got from this plan, was focus. In short, if you want to run five miles a day, you need to focus on running. If you want to lose a pound a day, you need to focus on weight loss!

I'll add here as a side note that research published in *Medicine & Science in Sports & Exercise* shows marathon running to be a very effective way to *maintain* one's desired weight once it is reached.[34] In other words, go ahead and get the running shoes on once you've hit your goal weight, but again, you may not want to confuse two goals, thinking that running to train for a marathon on a daily basis will bring you down into the weight range in which you desire to be.

Focus, in this way, can be applied in many areas of our lives. *Focus is everything.* If you want to do anything, you need to focus on it. A great mentor of mine, Ann Bolger, told me that in order to accomplish my goals, I'd sometimes need to be like a horse wearing blinders, focused only on what was ahead, without distraction.[35] This applies to so many areas!

If you want to write a book, you need to get extremely focused on writing, editing, and publishing that book. If you want to be a great video gamer, you're going to need to spend a lot of time gaming. You cannot get good at a video game if you keep stopping to write paragraphs for your book, and you cannot get good at writing books if you spend hours playing video games. If you want to learn an instrument, spend time learning that instrument. If you want to get good grades, focus on getting good grades. There are so many distractions that come up in life. Too many of us take on too much at once and never truly accomplish our goals because we are not focused. It gets worse:

We often can be distracted from the activities that will bring us further toward our goals, by activities that *seem* productive!

If you're trying to be a great concert violinist, yet you spend all of your time exercising, you may never accomplish your most important goal! Though you and others may find your exercising to *seem* productive (who would balk at exercise?), if overdone, it may not align with your ultimate intentions and may end up detracting from your ability to be successful at learning the violin. I'm not saying that a violinist shouldn't exercise. What I'm saying is that too much exercise could detract from time spent improving at the violin and may ultimately lead to mediocrity in both areas.

If you allow yourself to be distracted, even by activities that others would consider to be productive, and those activities distract you from your goal, you will fail at that goal.

As Bill Phillips, brilliant entrepreneur and author of *Body for Life*, said about goals, "Half of getting what you want is knowing what you have to give up to get it."[36]

This may seem simple, but it's important: If you want to lose weight, you need to *focus* on losing weight. You need to take a very direct, focused approach to do what it takes to lose weight, if that is your goal.

Looking back, I had actually been sacrificing valuable resting and cooking time by straining my body too much with exercise. While it was most in need of rest and proper nutrition, my body was getting sleep deprivation and constant stressful exertion.

That never worked well for me, and now I understand it much better. Now, if given spare time in a day, I will first use it to cook meals, then to make sure I am well rested and that I have stocked up on healthy groceries. Then, if I still have time available in that day, I'll go for a run or hit the weights. I feel like I had it upside-down before and prioritized exercise over things like healthy eating and sleep, which I now know to be very important to my well-being. I'll also mention that now, at over 30 pounds lighter, I can *fly* when I'm outside running!

So, for Phase 2, don't feel like you're missing out when you go for a few weeks without hitting the gym, as long as that's what your healthcare professionals have prescribed. Enjoy the downtime, and learn to live a life with good nutrition. The exercise will come later in Phases 3 and 4.

HCG AND YOUR HEALTH

BY NOW YOU'RE THINKING, *Wait, no exercise, and injections – this must be bad for you!* Get this. My pre-HCG blood pressure was 133 over 84. It was high – way too high for my age and way too high for someone with no family history of high blood pressure. I wasn't alone. The Center for Disease Control (CDC) reports that 67 million American adults (31%) have high blood pressure—that's 1 in every 3 adults. Only about half (47%) of people with high blood pressure have their condition under control.[37] I wasn't just overweight, I was unhealthy. My motivation for my transformation was not to bring down my blood pressure, but when I found out after losing the 30 pounds that it had dropped to 109 over 75, I was genuinely happier about that part of my results than about any other piece, including my baggier jeans.

I couldn't believe how much my blood pressure had changed due to my healthy eating! It was amazing! My initial reason for doing this was because I wanted to look and feel better and be able to fit into my clothes again. But when it came down to it, the thing that made me that happiest after all was said and done was that drop in blood pressure – I'd done something to truly make myself healthier, and that felt great.

It gets better. While on the HCG diet, I needed to cook vegetables and meats constantly. As I mentioned, my nutritionist wouldn't allow me to eat foods like lunch meat, which is full of preservatives. I had only one choice, which was to cook things myself. I also needed a way to get lots of vegetables into my system, so I was forced to shop a lot more than I had before. I had to find vegetables and find ways to prepare them so that Derrick would actually eat them when he got hungry. After spending so much time preparing foods, I learned how to eat healthy! After Phase 2 was complete, I was excited to be able to eat more of the same, healthy foods. To this day, I'm constantly using my time to cook various foods that are nutritious and that I really like to eat. I now even favor healthier choices when I go to restaurants.

What I am telling you is that my tastes have actually changed.

Don't get me wrong – my tastes have not changed like those veggie-loving, smoothie-drinking movie people say they will. I'm not eating a pile of kale anytime in the near future. I'm sure that's possible, but I'm not there just yet. That's for another time and another book.

Having said that, I'm now much more likely to order vegetables at a great restaurant or mix in some onions, peppers, tomatoes, and mushrooms into foods. As I've mentioned, the research backs why I'm doing this. A 2013 *Appetite* journal article reported that weight loss leads to a reduction in craving of harmful, fatty foods.[38]

It gets even better! As I'll discuss later in the book, the drinks I used to enjoy like gin and tonics tasted seemed to have a "poison" taste after my weight loss period. This poison taste was more apparent immediately after my program, and is now still there, but to a lesser extent. I drink very little hard liquor now, and one of my favorite drinks used to be the gin and tonic. I used to enjoy beer if I was out with friends, and now when I drink it I feel like I'm taking down a glass of sugar for no reason. I actually now favor red wine and have begun to choose it over other options. I didn't give up alcohol entirely, and there's even actually research showing that in moderation it can be healthy. Harvard Medical School published that there is solid evidence that alcohol in moderation offers some protection against heart disease and ischemic (clot-caused) stroke and that it probably reduces premature deaths in healthy people as well as those with diabetes, and high blood pressure.[39] I now just drink less than I used to. I think part of that is because my tastes have changed, and a bigger part of that is because I've found through this transition that I have so much more to do, and so little time to distract myself with that kind of downtime. I'm thankful that I've been able to find more balance through this transition.

My tastes have shifted in such a way that I'll naturally live a healthier lifestyle, and it's because I did this HCG diet.

I also want to mention that I learned a lot about how my body reacts to different foods. I now know how chicken with grilled peppers makes me feel, as compared to a bowl of pasta or a candy bar. If I'm feeling down, I can now pinpoint – often to the meal – when I ate the thing that caused my physiology to change and create a mood that I normally wouldn't have. I'm very aware of how foods affect my body and I'm constantly making active decisions about what to eat in order to have the right mindset later in the day. My digestion is better than ever, and my energy levels are so high that I wrote and published a *whole damn book* (that you're now reading).

Finally, my favorite part about all of this is that I now feel like I am truly in the driver's seat when it comes to my weight. There are two things that used to happen when I would lose weight. First, I would worry when I gained three or four pounds back, because I would think it was an uncontrollable cycle and that I was going to "gain it *all* back." Second, I actually would not worry *enough* when I gained just a pound or two because I felt it was just "water weight." I now do two things much differently. When I gain a pound or two, I don't "worry," yet am *very* conscious of it, and I react immediately and effectively to control it. I almost never let myself get as far as a three pound gain, because by the time I'm up two pounds, it's recognized and under control.

Research published in the *British Journal of Health Psychology* supports this strategy, showing that successful weight maintainers adopt a staged approach to weight management, including monitoring weight fluctuations and having a clear alarm signal for weight gain that triggers immediate action. The same research shows that these successful weight maintainers have several behavioral strategies for weight control, comprising relatively small adjustments to diet and/or exercise behavior and also have clear strategies for coping with lifestyle interruptions.[40]

Research from the *Journal of Behavioral Medicine* also supports this approach, indicating that that self-regulatory skills training might actually be just as effective as dietary and physical activity advice in terms of weight loss![41] Because I monitor my weight so closely, and have developed the strategies you're reading right here, when I face a challenge, I am in control and immediately capable of bringing my weight back down to the point where I know it should be. I now do not fluctuate as much in weight, regardless of what I eat. As I'll discuss later in this book, my body has also achieved a "set point," where it seems more difficult for my weight to break out of its new range, making it easier to maintain this weight.

This all started because of a small period of time when I used HCG to lose weight.

I included this chapter because I hear constant criticism of weight loss strategies that include this level of calorie restriction and this magnitude of rapid weight loss. Yet, I have gained so many healthy habits from this change, that my experience would be very hard to characterize as unhealthy. If my new habits sound healthy to you, I agree, because I sure feel healthier. For me, fast weight loss led to lower blood pressure, new habits, and sustainable patterns, that research shows will carry me forward at a healthy weight. Remember, I was injecting the HCG hormone for a limited period of about five weeks. The rest of this thinking and acting has become a part of my daily life, and will last for years to come.

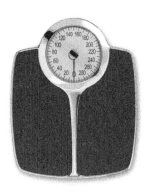

PART 3:
BEFORE YOU START YOUR
PROGRAM

PART 3 IS A collection of the best advice I can give you about preparing to start your program. After reading this, you may find that you're not ready to start, and that's a good discovery to make before you waste your time! You shouldn't start a program until you're ready. Use this next section of the book to guide you in that decision.

BEFORE YOU START: BE READY TO COMMIT

CHOOSING WHEN TO START your plan is an essential part of success. If you pick a time that is full of tempting events or is highly stressful, you may be destined to fail. On the other side of that coin, if you are strategic about picking a time to start this plan, it can help you! A big part of my advice is knowing yourself and your surroundings. If you can find ways to use your own habits or your surroundings to your advantage, your chances of success skyrocket.

I chose to start my weight loss plan at a time when most people would not: the holidays. I was headed into the Thanksgiving and Christmas season, when a lot of family events and vacations tend to occur and when people are bringing lots of treats into the office. Some would say that this was the worst time to start such a plan, but for me, it ended up being highly advantageous. Here's why.

The holidays are a time when people tend to have a lot going on. They need to shop, they need to spend time with their families, and they need to go to lots of parties. For that reason, the holidays can sometimes be less stressful when it comes to work itself. I found that my job was not as demanding in the November to December timeframe as usual, because most of the people I worked with were scattered about, trying to get things done. During that time, I was able to actually cut out of work earlier than I normally would. This was crucial, because during this time I needed to see my nutritionist once a week, while also spending a lot of time cooking healthy foods. Because I chose a time when work wasn't stressful, I was able to spend more time out of the office. I found efficiencies by doing my Christmas shopping online, and I used the spare time that everyone else spent scurrying about town to cook healthy pieces of chicken and to grill asparagus.

I also chose a good time to start my weight loss plan because one of my worst influences (and close friends) would be out of town. To protect the innocent, let's call my friend Commodore Longfellow. Commodore Longfellow is one of the most bright, fun people in the world to be around. Commodore Longfellow also eats more junk food than any human being I've ever met. Specifically, I have seen him walk into a meeting with a two-liter of Pepsi and two bags of chips and eat it all right in front of the group. Commodore Longfellow is massive in stature, standing a full six feet, six inches. Commodore Longfellow will not only invite you to come to the bar after work, but he will humiliate you if you say you won't go. He will tell you that you are "lame" and that you are "boring" and that you are going to "go home and cry yourself to sleep." He will make fun of your diet and your food choices and he will tell you that you will "gain it all back." Commodore Longfellow is one of my best friends, but at times it seems there is no changing him, and he is absolutely one of the worst people to have around you while you are trying to lose weight, because he will try his best to sabotage your plan. He honestly, in his heart of hearts, believes that you are an idiot for trying to be healthier, and he communicates this clearly.

There may be a Commodore Longfellow in your life, and if there is, I suggest this: Find a time when you can get yourself away from your Commodore Longfellow for about a month and use that time to start losing weight. In my case, I was able to find a time when Commodore Longfellow would be traveling for business for most of the low-calorie, HCG Phase 2 period. I used this time to my advantage. By the time Commodore Longfellow was back in the area, I was already a good 20 pounds lighter and nearly headed into my maintenance phases.

You should probably also think about picking a time to start when you won't be bogged down by heavy projects at work or at home. If you have a lot going on and you're working to meet deadlines, it's likely that during Phase 2, you won't be able to find the discipline to head home early and make sure you're in bed before you get hungry and start eating. This is a short period of time when you will need to be very focused on eating the right things. If there are a lot of distractions in your life, it is not a good time to get this program going.

I know someone who tried starting the HCG plan when the time wasn't right for him.

Two weeks after he started his plan, I asked him how he was progressing. He immediately gave me a set of excuses about how he was too busy. He had participated in a couple of obligatory social events over the weekend and felt he needed to eat a lot and drink alcohol while he was there.

My first thought when I heard this was, *What's wrong with this guy?* Then I realized that there was nothing wrong – and that was the problem! The problem was that he wasn't dissatisfied enough yet. He didn't really, really want to change. He just wasn't ready.

Everyone is busy. Everyone has events. I made my transformation while pursuing a graduate degree, during the holiday season (including Thanksgiving), while I took vacations and worked 50 hours per week. We all have obligations. We're all busy. If you're making excuses, it's because you're not ready for this yet. That's fine, but just don't start it until you're ready. I'll say it again…

Don't start until you're ready.

There *is* a way to be successful, no matter where you are, who you are, and what you're doing, but it requires that you're prepared, that you take very real steps to make sure you're prepared, that you have a burning desire, and that you follow a plan. I will talk more about this later, but I will say now that if you intend to start this program thinking, *Hopefully I will lose some weight,* you will fail. You need to pick a time when you are highly free of distraction and highly motivated to do this.

BEFORE YOU START: GETTING SPECIFIC ABOUT YOUR BURNING DESIRE

HERE'S SOME IMPORTANT ADVICE you've probably heard in many languages.

If you want to make a change, you need to have a reason.

Sounds simple, right? The thing is, the reason needs to be a burning reason. It can't just be you saying to yourself, *Oh, I'd like to just be a little bit skinnier.* If even a part of you is okay with where your physique is today, then it's going to be very difficult for you to stay motivated to create *massive* change in your life! You need to have a burning desire to change, and once that desire exists, you'll be able to find the tools to change it. Where there's a will, there's a way, as you've heard many times before.

This is the most important thing you will read in this book, and it is the key to losing weight or doing anything in life. If you want to create lasting change, in any way, you need to have a deep, burning desire to create that change.

This desire needs to be so strong that it wakes you up earlier than usual so you're excited to jump on the scale. It needs to be a desire so strong that it makes you laugh in the face of temptation. This desire to change needs to burn so deep that you don't even *want* that piece of birthday cake because you've grown to hate your unhealthy life and the result it has had on your lifestyle. If you don't have that level of desire – or you had it and it has gone away – you cannot create the change you need to in order to be successful.

You need to complete a very sincere self-inventory before you decide to make any big change. Do you really, really care about making change in your life? Do you really, really care? Really, really think about this. If your answers are, "I'll see how I feel," or, "I won't really go all-out, I'll just try my best," then you're not where you need to be in order to make a successful change. No hormone, meal plan, or supplement, whether it's HCG, juicing, cabbage soup, or lemon juice, can help you or anyone who doesn't choose to live a different life and truly make a change. You need to be willing to do whatever it takes; then – and only then – you will be ready to be successful.

There may be a placebo for HCG. There is no placebo for burning desire.

Think about it. You're about to embark on a plan in which you can only eat about 500 calories of food per day. That's next to nothing! If you are at all happy with your current physique, you aren't mad enough to do this. If that's the case, go for a run or sign up for a Zumba class! Don't inject yourself with stuff every morning if you're not ready to commit!

If you are satisfied with how you feel and look, there is no way you can overcome the temptation you're about to face in this type of a plan. If you do not want to change, it will not work. If you are happy with where you are, it will not work.

I'll tell you how I learned this. To be honest, I have now done two cycles of HCG. The first, which I'm writing about in this book, worked beautifully. The second cycle did not work at all. Why didn't it work? I made the mistake of forgetting that my desire was much more important than my plan, yet I had no desire left. I was happy with my new weight, and trying to lose more was almost impossible, because I was not willing to give up the food to do it! I had been stable and delightedly happy in Phases 3 and 4 for months, and I was thinking that I would use my mad HCG skills to drop down to a very cut weight, 30 pounds lower than my initial goal weight. See, I had always *wanted* abs (who doesn't, right?), but I realized that I wouldn't give anything up to get there. I didn't want them that bad. I didn't want them even one-millionth as bad as I had wanted to stop my belt from digging into my belly and be able to wear normal clothes back before all of this started. Once I had achieved my first set of goals, I didn't care enough about the ancillary goal of getting "ripped" in order to really pursue it. Maybe if I had a deep, burning desire to look like the guys on the covers of magazines, I would have been able to take the steps needed to do that. I just don't.

The problem (and this will sound funny) was that I was happy!

I was very happy with my new weight and my new appearance. I didn't need any more weight loss, and I wasn't willing to put in the hard work that I had once been willing to put in, because I'd reached a state of satisfaction. So what did I do during that second cycle? I started to eat less methodically. I didn't even eat as well during my second round of Phase 2 as I had been eating for the last three months on Phases 3 and 4! On Phases 3 and 4, I had been preparing very healthy foods and enjoying them all day. In Phase 2, I had to cut my caloric intake so low that I'd end up eating a larger meal at night, because I was very hungry, yet I was happy with what I saw in the mirror! I realized I had no burning desire to go beyond what I'd accomplished, and fighting through hunger just wasn't worth it anymore. I decided after a matter of days to return to healthily eating foods from Phase 4 to continue to maintain my previous weight.

Learn from my failure here. You need to have a burning desire to lose the weight, and that desire has to be your own. It cannot be your family's desire, or your friend's or anyone else's. It has to be your reason, your vision, and it has to burn so hot and bright that you'll do whatever it takes to get there. If you don't have that, lend this book to a friend or shelf it until you do. Come back with the desire, and we can work together.

Mothers tell their children that they can be anything they want to be in life. To some extent, I think that's true. To some extent, I think it's not.

I do not believe that you can do anything that you simply *want* to do; however, I *strongly* believe that you can achieve anything if you have an *undying passion* that burns so deep in your soul that you would give anything to get there.

You need to want something so bad that you will either succeed at getting it or die trying.

Yoda said it best: "There is no try, only do."

He could have been talking about HCG there. This plan isn't worth trying. It's only worth doing.

Read Napoleon Hill's book, *Think and Grow Rich*, and you'll find that the author hides the secret of accomplishing anything within its pages.[42] My summary of his secret is this: Be willing to die trying.

Tony Robbins, the great motivator, tells his readers that the only way to achieve something is to be motivated by both the intense feeling of pain that you want to avoid, and toward the great feeling of pleasure you want to achieve.[43] If you can't yet feel that pain on a deep level or envision that pleasure with the same intensity, *you aren't ready*!

The sad truth is that many people aren't willing to do what it takes to get to where they want to be. A great leader and close friend of mine often used to tell me, "Everyone wants to go to heaven, but nobody wants to die to get there."

Rich Roll, an ultra-marathoner who has been proclaimed one of the fittest men in the world by Men's Fitness magazine[44] and the author of *Finding Ultra*,[45] writes a fantastic blog. In one of his posts, he interviewed the talented film director Casey Neistat, who relayed what he referred to as a "recipe for success he guarantees to work." Neistat said,

"All you have to do is commit your entire life to something, which will result in one of two outcomes. Either you will succeed, or you will die trying, which is in and of itself its own form of success."[46]

I would venture to bet that there are very few accidental millionaires. There are absolutely no accidental doctors or lawyers or Ph.Ds. There are no accidental Everest summiteers or marathon finishers. All of these people have something in common. They were all willing to give up almost everything in life – sometimes including life itself – to achieve something. This desire created the commitment that enabled them to get through the months and years of agony that led to their ultimate accomplishment.

So you want to be healthy? You want to be lighter? Skinnier? Are you willing to give up alcohol? Are you willing to give up the feeling of being full of food? Are you willing to give up your social life for a little while? Are you willing to part ways with a friend, or maybe even a significant other, who holds you back or who is a bad influence? Are you willing to give up the tastes of some of your favorite foods for a few months? Do you want it that badly?

Do you want it that badly?

Give yourself an honest answer here. If it's "yes," I'll see you in the next chapter.

BEFORE YOU START:
DON'T BE A WEASEL

"Weaseling out of things is important to learn. It's what separates us from the animals! Except the weasel."
-Homer Simpson

WE'VE TALKED ABOUT THE HCG plan being highly prescriptive and about how that is beneficial. Now, before we go any further, I want to share something with you that will be critical to your success if you choose to try this or any prescriptive program.

If your nutritionist's advice is, "Don't drink zero-calorie soft drinks," you don't drink them. **You don't drink them.** *You don't drink them.* When your nutritionist says not to drink zero-calorie soft drinks, DO NOT try to find one that's okay. DO NOT try to propose other options. You just don't do it. You ask that nutritionist what to drink, and she will tell you, and you will drink it. That's that.

If your nutritionist tells you not to use lotion that contains oils, you don't do it. Just don't. Don't question it. Don't say, "That doesn't sound right." You listen to your nutritionist and you do what she says. You throw away those lotions and you go lotion-less.

Do you see a pattern here?

You do whatever it is that your team of healthcare professionals tells you to do. Period. If you do this, you will succeed. If you don't, you will probably fail.

I did exactly what my nutritionist told me to do and exactly what she wrote down, and I succeeded. It was that simple. If you're being a weasel, you're not ready to commit at the level you need to.

So many people I talk to about their diet are thinking the wrong way. Right away, they're thinking of ways to cheat themselves. If you tell them they can't have meat, right away they'll ask, "Can I have a little turkey?" If you tell them not to have sugar, they'll ask, "Can I have sugar-free candy?" They're being weasels. Don't be one of them.

In the past, a nutritionist told me that I needed to start cooking, and, being a weasel, I immediately started to find ways that I could buy pre-cooked meats. At the time, I lost almost no weight. I was a weasel. When I stopped being a weasel and started listening (and therefore cooking), I got immediate results.

If you're going to be that guy or gal who just can't seem to understand that you need to change your ways in order to change your life, then it's not going to work for you.

You need to wake up, grab yourself by the love handles (literally do this regularly – I honestly recommend it as a good reminder of your progress) and understand that if you want to make a change for the better, what you've been doing won't work anymore. You need to give your actions over to someone else for a while so that you can learn how to do something new.

Do what they say. Do what they say.
Do what they say.

Follow the prescription. Don't try to think up ways to cheat. Don't be a weasel.

BEFORE YOU START: WRITING DOWN YOUR REASONS

RESEARCH PUBLISHED IN THE *Western Journal of Nursing Research* shows that a significant turning point leads to an identity shift in people who are able to lose weight and keep it off.[47] I advise you to define this turning point, by writing down all of the reasons you need to change, right now.

As I set out on this plan, I sat down and wrote what it was that I truly hated about my life. Notice, I'm not saying *what I disliked* or *what I found to be inconvenient*. I'm using *hate*, which is a very strong word, for a reason. I had grown to truly hate a few things and I wrote them down so that I could look back as I made progress or ran into hurdles, so that I could better remember the pain that I was moving away from.

Your reasons for initiating change in your life have to be *yours*, and they have to form a *burning desire*. Whatever they are, write them down! These will be your reminders of why you need to continue when you face adversity. My written reasons included topics that were all across the board. They included things like not being able to wear my polo shirts because they were too tight and having my aforementioned belt-mark. They included my double chin in pictures, not being able to wear my suits, and the pain I would experience when I would have to sit all day at work in pants that were too small for me. These may seem silly to you, or maybe they don't. Regardless, these were *my* reasons – *my* reminders of pain – that I needed to be very in-touch with in order to be successful. I looked at this list *daily* as I progressed. I believe a great part of my success was due to this list.

You need to make a list of the reasons you *hate* this aspect of your life.

That may sound harsh to you, and I'm okay with being harsh right now because I'm here to help you, and because you can't slap me from where you're sitting. In any area of your life, if you're mainly satisfied with things the way they are, I believe it's going to be very difficult for you to take the steps necessary to get those things to change.

I also made a list of the things I had to look forward to, in exchange for my current sacrifice. For me, these included being able to wear t-shirts again (I couldn't wear them at the time, because I felt too chubby in them), being able to go to the pool without being embarrassed, and being able to run long distances without hurting my knees. I looked forward to being more confident and less self-conscious. These things meant a lot to me, and I looked at this list every single day of my weight loss period, too. These things might mean nothing to you, and that's okay, because they were *my* reasons. You need to know yours.

Make a list of the reasons you need to succeed, painting the picture of what it will be like when you get there.

Finally, I made a list of my absolute goals, and I wrote them out in a very visual manner. These included the actual weight I wanted to arrive at by the end of my weight loss in Phase 2. They included a purchase I'd always wanted as a reward for my accomplishment, and as a way to remember what it took to achieve my goal. My goals included going home to visit my family at Christmas and having a happier demeanor than I usually had, because for the first time in years, I would be less chubby and more proud of who I'd become.

Again, for you, these goals might not hit home, because they're not yours. You need to write down your specific goals for your transformation. Research published in *Clinical Rehabilitation* shows that writing down specific, measurable, achievable, realistic / relevant, and timed goals (a process called SMART) is useful in goal attainment.[48] Moreover, in a research study published in the *Journal of Experimental Social Psychology*, participants were tracked over the course of a 12-week weight loss program that directed participants' focus toward their end weight loss goal or toward what they had already achieved. Goal-focused participants reported higher levels of commitment to their goal and, ultimately, lost more weight than did no focus control participants![49] Set goals.

Make a very specific list of what you want to accomplish and even how you'll reward yourself. Write down how you'll feel as well.

As embarrassing as it is to write down the things above, being transparent about my life like this, I believe I need to do it so that you can understand how specific you need to get with your writing. To you, this stuff might just make you chuckle or think I'm a bit petty, but petty or not, the whole point is that these are the real things that *moved* me to the extent I was willing to make massive changes in my day-to-day life.

What are the things that move you? If you can't write them down, you won't be able to get through the rough waters.

If you can clearly see what's ahead, what you're leaving behind, and you understand what you'll need to sacrifice to get to where you want to be, your chances of success will be much greater.

Make your own list before you even start down this path. It's not worth trying to move forward until you understand why you're doing it.

BEFORE YOU START: "JUMPER CABLES"

I'VE BEEN KNOWN TO conduct a presentation on goal-setting that I believe may help you a bit here. In this presentation I discuss the concept of "jumper cables." You're already probably very familiar with the jumper cables that are used to restart a car when the battery is dead. What I'm referring to here are "mental" jumper cables.

Here's what I mean.

Mental jumper cables are a way to get you back on track when your motivation is zapped and you can't seem to overcome your temptations. They're a way to immediately change your mental state and get you back on the right path when you face adversity.

To create these mental jumper cables, I want you to think about your goal and I want you to think about the worst pain you've ever come across, related to that goal. Has there been a time when you were too under-confident to ask someone on a date because of your weight? Worse, has someone actually rejected you for that reason? Use it. Remember it. Is there an outfit or a certain item you couldn't wear because of your size? Use that too. Dr. Scott Lewis tells us, "Everyone has that one outfit that they truly love that doesn't fit so well anymore. Often times, when we outgrow these beloved garments through weight gain, these outfits, whether they're a slim fitting dress or a tailored suit, end up crammed in the very back of the closet, in the dark. They are left unused, as they can feel like shameful reminders of the size you used to be. But guess what: that is the exact opposite of what you should be doing with them. They're ignored and useless when they're left in the back of the closet. Instead, it's time to bring them out of the darkness and use them as motivational tools. Keep them in front so you want to fit in to them again. Visualize yourself in them, and once you reach your goal, wear these items out, and reap the rewards of all of your hard work."[50]

Now is the time to be very real about what it is that emotionally grips you and makes you feel terrible, then *use that* to your advantage. Whatever it is, it needs to be *your* pain and nobody else's. Write it down, and be descriptive.

Now, related to that same goal, I want you to think about the most positive aspects of accomplishing this goal. What are the most compelling reasons to make this happen? Visualize your life when you're 30, 60, or 90 pounds lighter. What are you wearing? What are you doing? Who are you with? Why is life better? Whatever those burning desires are, get them on paper.

Now, take the pain and the pleasure and make sure those written, vivid statements are right there with you. Some people even choose to make "vision boards" out of them, with cutouts from magazines allowing them to visualize the future. Whatever it may be, grab it, make it a physical artifact, and carry it or make it readily accessible on your smartphone or laptop.

You now have your "jumper cables." Visualize these things as often as you can – daily, or hourly if you can make the time. Make them so ingrained into your memory that you can't help but think about them and, more importantly, experience the emotions that accompany them. Then, use that! When temptation sets in and you feel like your "battery is dead," think of those things! Bring yourself back to re-experiencing that pain and that pleasure and do it again and again in your mind until the chocolates in front of you are something you can just toss to the side.

I suggest you use this and other techniques to increase and maintain your levels of motivation. Research actually has proven that higher levels of sustained and learned motivation are associated with higher rates of weight loss.[51] In my experience, this technique can be powerful if applied correctly, and though it may not be as high-impact as waking yourself up at 4:00 A.M., it's certainly worth trying.

BEFORE YOU START:
SET YOUR ALARM CLOCK

WE'VE TALKED NOW ABOUT knowing yourself, and I shared with you one of my favorite tips, which is to wake up really early while you're trying to lose weight. I absolutely know that this was a major factor in my success in this program. My advice to you, if you struggle with late-night binging as I did, is to get up as early as you possibly, humanly can.

I advise this for two reasons. First, because if you get up early, you get tired and go to bed early. Second, because if you're anything like me or most people I know well, you are much less likely to binge on unhealthy food and alcohol early in the morning than you are late at night. In my experience, there are very few people in this world who get out of bed in the morning and start binging on pizzas and beer. There are very few people who roll out of bed and head to a bar and overdo it. (If you're a morning binger, you may want to reverse this advice.) Fred Turek, director of the Center for Sleep and Circadian Biology at Northwestern University says that late-night eating may be worse, in terms of weight gain, than eating during normal waking hours.[52]

For these reasons, I get up now at 4:00 A.M. almost every day. During my weight loss, no matter what, I would force myself out of bed that early. I now may sleep until about 6:00 A.M. at the latest, but that's a rare event. I'll explain in detail.

Whether you consider yourself a morning person or not, a high-impact way to make this happen is to force yourself to wake up as early as you can, every day, and not take a nap. Trust me, you'll end up going to bed earlier after a few days of this repeated behavior.

Take keen notice that my advice was not "go to bed earlier." You can tell yourself to do that all you want, but you're not going to do that. Why? *Because your body isn't used to it. Because you didn't wake up earlier. You're not going to be tired.* If you tell yourself to go to bed earlier, your body won't listen. (Remember the part about getting to know yourself?)

Instead of trying to will yourself to sleep, I recommend that you set that alarm for 4:00 A.M., force yourself out of bed when the alarm goes off, and grab some coffee or green tea instantly. Drink up while being lazy and watching TV or whatever you want to do until it kicks in at 5:20 or so. When it kicks in and you're ready to face the world, that's when it's time to be productive. If you're not on HCG, then you may choose for this to be your time to work out. If you're on HCG, I suggest using this time to do some journaling and prepare food for the day.

Having said all of this, let me be clear about something.

Even if you wake up this early and you do absolutely nothing but waste time and watch TV, it was worth it.

You are waking up this early, not because you need to use the time productively *now*, but because you are ensuring you'll be able to sleep when 9:00 or 10:00 P.M. rolls around. Some mornings, I would get up and watch two hours of television without doing anything else productive.

I was happy with this result! That's because there are two things I wasn't going to do. One, binge on food, and two, stay up late that night. The fact of the matter is, I ended up being more productive just because I was up early. Establishing this new habit is what allowed me to write this book! I found that about two-thirds of the mornings, I'd get up tired and just cook food for the day (another plus) and not do much else. About one-third of the time, I'd be extremely productive, either writing a chapter of this book or getting a workout in.

The big benefits to getting up early like this are that you get prep time for food, you don't end up binging, and you don't end up staying up late and overeating or drinking. The ancillary benefit is that you sometimes won't be able to help yourself – you'll actually just start getting things done in the morning. Also, if you have a flexible work schedule and you can get into the office just an hour or so earlier, it feels really good to be done with the workday early and get out while there's still daylight. I'm not trying to get you to fit more into your day here. I'm trying to get you to *shift* your day so that you're awake during your most productive and least "binge-y" hours and asleep during your least productive and most "binge-y" hours. I'm trying to get you to use the fact that you know yourself!

I'll amplify here, as I said before, that on weekends, you still should be waking up this early. If you don't, you're much more likely to stay up late at night and possibly do things that could lead to weight gain. Also, you will throw off your cycle for the rest of the week. On weekends, you still want to be tired at 9:00 P.M. Sure, you won't be able to hang out with friends until late into the evening or stay up late enough to watch *Saturday Night Live*. If you're a late-night eater, you're just going to need to make sacrifices in order to use this method of adaptation. Research published in the *International Journal of Obesity & Related Metabolic Disorders* backs this concept, showing that people who are able to maintain their healthy eating habits across a full week (including weekends) will have better success maintaining them across the year – including vacations and holidays.[53] Go ahead and relax on the weekends, just get up early to do it! Remember, using this system, you get as much time as anyone else does in the day, you just get your free time in the morning instead of at night.

I can say from having done this for months that I have just as much fun watching movies in the morning as I did watching movies at night.

In conclusion, if you tend to snack at night, try not being up at night.

As an afterthought, I really started to enjoy this time in the morning. I'm still, to this day, excited to get up and face the day as a healthier person. I like sitting with my coffee before the sun rises, even if I'm just watching TV and planning for the day. I wrote this very paragraph at 5:20 A.M.!

Now, for those of you saying, "I'm not a morning person," I think that with a will behind it, you have more control over that than you think. If you moved to India, and your schedule needed to change by over twelve hours, could you figure it out? I believe you could.

Having said that, I started all of this with, "Know thyself." This remains true. If you are different than me, that's of course, just fine.

Do what works for you based on what you know your past habits to be.

Don't take advice from me if it doesn't fit your life. Use what you know about yourself to make a plan work for you. This one just worked for me and it worked really well, so I'm confident about sharing it.

If I still don't have you convinced, take the advice from Sallie Krawcheck, former head of Merrill Lynch and Smith Barney, as she wrote for LinkedIn Influencers.[54] In this article, Krawchek described waking up at 4:00 A.M., brewing a cup of coffee, keeping the lights down low, and feeling the sense of peace knowing that her family was safe upstairs as she was working. I agree with Sallie K. on this one – that time of the morning can be the best time of the day and, based on my results, can also save you from destroying your weight loss transformation with bad habits.

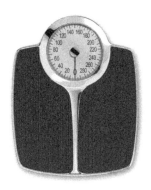

PART 4:
MY TRANSFORMATION,
WEEK BY WEEK

PART 4 IS A week-by-week account of my transformation during this program. Use this as a guide and allow me to be your partner as you progress!

BEFORE THE WEIGHT LOSS: NOT RECOGNIZING MYSELF AND PROBLEMS WITH JEANS

IN THE MONTHS LEADING up to my decision to lose weight, a few things happened to me that you might be able to relate to. First, I realized that my clothes were stretched much tighter across certain areas of my body than they used to be. My button-down shirts, which used to hang loosely, were form-fitting and stretched tightly across my chest.

My belt buckle, which never had seemed problematic before, had started to poke into the underside of my belly, causing a red mark there that never seemed to go away. On top of this, I was sweating too much and too often.

In pictures, I was almost unrecognizable to myself. When I looked in the mirror, I still saw the same guy who I'd always seen there. But in pictures, every angle seemed to be a bad one! I just wasn't looking like "me," and it was a bit surreal.

I went to the store to get some jeans. I always buy my jeans at the same store, because their jeans are insanely comfortable and the people at the store serve you beer while you try them on. The jeans there happen to be on the expensive side. Say what you want about that store. Call me elitist, because those jeans are costly, but you know what? They're beyond comfortable. It's like I'm wearing pajamas all day, but it's socially acceptable. I love them. I buy about two pairs of them per year, and they're what I wear almost every single day. I figure if you're going to spend a lot of money, spend it on something you'll use all the time. Save money on things you use repeatedly for a few seconds, and where quality doesn't matter as much. Spend as much as you can afford on things like your couch – which you have to sit on for the next twenty years – or your refrigerator or pens. Okay, I get that pens are something that you use for a relatively short time, but a good pen that writes well is just heavenly, isn't it? Just heavenly, a good pen can be. Your priorities will be different from mine. I just suggest that you invest in long-term purchases, and save on things you'll forget you bought by tomorrow morning!

Back to jeans. When I buy jeans, I always buy the same size. When you buy this certain brand of jeans, they're really tight until you wash them a few times, and then they loosen up. This time, I tried them on, and they were ultra-tight, but, like always, I bought them and took them home to wash them. I thought that, as usual, I would break them in and start including them in my man-rotation (meaning that I planned to wear them almost daily because even if people noticed the repetition, they would never say anything). I followed the usual drill, but this time, even after break-in, they were still too damn tight. In fact, they were unwearable. I put them on and felt like I had switched pants with a schoolboy (I realize that nobody uses the word schoolboy anymore, but I do because I find it funny). You get the point. The jeans were small. *Or I was big.*

It was this – and a few other key moments – that got me to realize I really had gotten bigger than I ever had been in my life. Not to mention, I had just spent a small fortune on jeans that I could not wear and could not return after this aforementioned break-in period. I damn well was going to wear these jeans and I was not going to spend another fortune to get a bigger size. There was no way I was going up a size. So I went with the only other alternative. I was finally fed up and I was going to lose the weight. I got pissed off – pissed off enough to actually decide to make a change. *It was a critical moment. It was a turning point.*

HOW I FOUND HCG,
AND A BIT ON HABIT CHANGING

LET'S TAKE THIS ALL the way back to where we left off, shopping for jeans.

My jeans didn't fit. I felt the worst I had in my entire life and I was looking for a solution.

Before this program I had many ups and downs with my weight. I was an aspiring mountaineer and had accomplished two successful guided summits of Mt. Rainier and a one-day ascent and descent of Mt. Whitney. These mountains aren't anything like the Himalaya, but Rainier is as close as you can get without heading to Alaska or leaving the continent, and it requires a lot of physical training to climb successfully and safely. In the past, training to climb a mountain would always get me scared enough to fast (like – not eat) and slim down to a weight where at least I would not be a danger to my rope team (people tied to me with a rope). However, I had never done this in a healthy way by ingesting more of the right foods. Instead, I had done it by fasting and overtraining within overly limited timeframes. I never stayed at my climbing weight for long, and after a climb I would always rebound and get heavy due to my unhealthy habits.

A few months before starting this program, I decided to do this again, as usual. I was planning to select a mountain to climb, thereby scaring myself, and doing a lot of training and fasting the way I used to. I started down this path, but I quickly found that at my new age (I was no longer in my twenties) the fasting wasn't having the effect on my body that it used to. I could fast all I wanted and not drop a pound. I was just plain unhealthy and I found that what used to work wasn't going to work anymore.

Research supports my slump. Recent findings in the study of weight homeostasis have uncovered a host of hormones working to keep a stable healthy weight. When energy stores are depleted through dieting, over-compensation to replenish them often occurs. Overeating is one of the homeostatic responses.[55] In short, I needed a new answer if I was going to get to a healthy weight. Exercise, even lots of exercise, paired with a starvation diet, wouldn't do it.

The problem was that my metabolism was just plain slow, and I was eating junk. I wasn't overeating. As a matter of fact, I didn't have a sweet tooth, I almost never snacked. If anything, I would go all day at work without eating a thing, have a few drinks after work, and then have some pizza. My overall caloric intake wasn't even that high, but my body had gotten so used to not eating enough, while not doing anything, that it just wasn't burning anything at all. At one point in July, I was running every day, up to about five miles, and was actually gaining weight. In fact, I got up to an all-time personal high on the scale while I was running five miles per day!

I quickly came to terms with the fact that unless I learned and did something new, I was either going to get heavier or stay the same weight. I needed a new solution, which I found in HCG.

One day at work, I was wearing my tight jeans while teaching a class that focuses on the habits and communication styles that occur within great organizations. In that class I often use analogies and, when I discuss "identity," I bring up the analogy of someone who is trying to get healthy.

Dan Gilbert, founder of Quicken Loans and an all-around incredible man who's doing fantastic things to revive the city of Detroit, wrote:

"*What* we do is secondary to *who* we are."[56]

In my class, I talk about identity in the sense that it means more than actions do, because identity drives actions. *Habits* drive actions. Rodd Hairston, Chairman and CEO of Envision U, speaks about changing habits and argues that, by changing your habits, you eventually change your life.[57] By focusing on changing your habits, you ultimately form a new identity, and that identity carries you through life.

Think about it this way: If your habit is to get out of bed and smoke a cigarette, eventually that habit will cause you to become more and more unhealthy until you may eventually develop a smoking-related illness. But, if you can change that habit so that daily you get out of bed and do 20 pushups, then that habit will cause you to get stronger and stronger, for life. Form your habits and form your identity. Form your identity and change your life. Easier said than done, especially if your "Derrick" loves to smoke a cigarette in the morning!

In my class, I teach people that you can write a to-do list of all the things a healthy person does, go do all of those things, and still not become healthier, because your identity may make a thousand and one small decisions that inhibit your progress and that counteract the results of the good decisions you've made. Picture your to-do list for a "healthy you" right now. Say you write down a list that includes things healthy people do, like getting exercise, sufficient sleep, hydration, and good food. Even though you might check off all those things on your list on a daily basis, your identity – or your habits – still cause you to do other things that are counterproductive, like eating handfuls of candy during the day. You're going to miss your target, because even though you're doing the things that healthy people do, you're *ruining* your progress with the things that an unhealthy you (your "Derrick") still does. You get it.

Back to the class I was teaching. I used this fitness analogy, as I had many times before, asking the group, "What are the things that a healthy person does?"

One person raised her hand and said, "Visits a doctor." I added that to the list. Then I thought … *good point.*

Every single weight loss supplement and plan on the market seems to come with written instructions telling you to see a doctor if you're planning to start a weight loss program. The thing was (when it came to weight loss) I had never done it!

I thought, *I'm going to visit the damn doctor.* So I did. And that's how it all started.

THE FIRST VISIT TO THE DOCTOR

AFTER MAKING THE REALIZATION described above, I made an appointment with a doctor and went for a visit. I'm fortunate to have a doctor who is, quite literally, right across the street and also who is part of a clinic that focuses on overall health and staffs professionals including a nutritionist, a shrink (that's a technical term), and others who can help you to improve your overall health.

My doctor took my blood pressure, 133 over 84, and told me it was high – way too high for my age (34 at the time). I told him I was there to lose weight because I had man-boobs and a belly (I'm trying to give you the honest truth here, and I actually said these things). I asked him how best to do it. He said something very sensible that I mentioned earlier this book. My doctor told me that I should use whatever program I could stick to.

Be it Weight Watchers, some online diet, HCG, whatever – his advice was just pick something I could keep doing until I had reached a healthy weight. He also told me that I could see the nutritionist and that she could help me out, so I immediately scheduled an appointment.

The next day I went to the appointment with the in-house nutritionist, who listened to my explanation about my disdain for my general appearance and told me about the options I had. When she realized that I was pretty driven toward a goal, she let me know that if I wanted to really drop the weight, HCG could help me. I was determined, so I bought the biggest program they offered – a 12-week package including the HCG, weekly counseling, and all of the vitamins and supplements I needed. I weighed in that day at around 224 pounds on the doctor's scale.[58]

REALIZING I WAS OBESE

I FEEL THE NEED to comment at this point that I never thought of myself as someone who would use the HCG diet. I'd heard of it but I knew it required massive calorie restriction and injections, and I thought that was for obese people. In the past I might have been right about it not being for me. The difference was, I was now obese.

So many Americans are somewhat overweight that it has been easy for me to blend in at my office and out on the town. These days, blending in has nothing to do with health. It seems like now, if you blend in, it means you're unhealthy! Data show that the situation is worsening. Gallup surveys report that the adult obesity rate so far in 2013 is 27.2%, up from 26.2% in 2012, and is on pace to surpass all annual average obesity rates since Gallup-Healthways began tracking in 2008.[59] Look forward to plenty of commentary on that in a later chapter. In short, even though most people would have said I was "normal," I had become obese. It was a really sad time in my life, and I know that it's the same for many people. If you're reading this, you probably know what I mean when I talk about that feeling of, *How did I get here?* You look back and you may or may not be able to answer that question, but for some reason, you just kind of let yourself slip away. I think that realizing you've done that is an important first step.

One part of that first step for me was when my good friend Commodore Longfellow reminded me of my weight. In a conversation with Commodore Longfellow, I referred to myself as "a little overweight." Commodore Longfellow, the sensitive man he is, lost his composure laughing and said, "You're not overweight. You're fat." Honestly, before he said that, I never thought of myself as an obese person. But I was.

To give you a feel for it, I was floating between 219 and 224 pounds depending on when I weighed in, and I'm 5'11 ½" tall. (I have to give myself credit for that half-inch.)

To be in the healthy range, according to any chart you use, a man of my build and height should be between 160 and 175 pounds. There are different ways of measuring it, but any scientist you talk to would have called me unhealthy.

To give you perspective, as I sit here on belt notch seven after 30 pounds of weight loss, everyone calls me skinny, yet I can still grab a few inches of excess from my belly. Post-weight loss, I'm still considered overweight by the charts, and I'm still somewhat chubby and unhealthy, even though I can run a half-marathon at a reasonable pace. It's crazy, but as I mentioned, I still "fit in," and now people even tell me I'm skinny.

My whole point here is that I don't believe you should look around yourself to find out what "normal" is. These days, normal is unhealthy. Healthy is the new weird, and we need to be weird if we want to live to play with our grandkids, great-grandkids, and great-great-grandkids!

PHASE 1: BINGING AND SHARING THE NEWS

AS I MENTIONED, THE first two days on my HCG plan were "binge days." That means that I would get up in the morning, inject myself with HCG, and proceed to eat as much food as I possibly could all day. My nutritionist recommended pizza, ice cream, other starches, and anything I could pack in. The theory here is that you should eat as much as possible to make your metabolism more prepared to burn fat, and also lessen your risk of struggling with the significant calorie deficit you'll face during the first week of Phase 2. I'm glad I took the advice. In the end, it all worked out well.

The binging phase is hard, mainly because you've just committed to doing something to make drastic improvement in your life, and you're ready to go! At this point, you can't *wait* to get started with your weight loss, but instead, you have to spend two full days doing stuff you don't want to do in your life anymore! Even though you've been living a life full of binge days, you're ready to stop, and these two days are completely contradictory to your impulses at this point. Regardless, you have to do it, and it's gross.

So for the first two days, I went around just binging like crazy. At that point, I was attending a two-day conference for work, and so the people I was surrounded by were thinking I was pretty strange. They'd known me as someone who was typically a healthy eater, yet also someone who was a bit overweight. So it was interesting to them to see that I was packing food into my face.

I'd eat whatever I could get my hands on. At dinner on the first night, I ate fried chicken and I visited the salad bar to smother it in ranch dressing. I drank four beers. I tried all of the appetizers available at the restaurant we visited on night two. Because people understood that I was binging because of my start on the HCG diet, they were having fun by passing me their leftovers to see what I would eat. I was stuffed and couldn't breathe as they passed me ice cream, but I ate it. I did it all for a reason: I was turning my life over to a plan from my doctor and nutritionist that I believed in. I did everything I was supposed to. According to my journal, I went from 220 pounds on the first day to 222.5 pounds two days later. That's surprisingly little gain for someone who did what I did. I even ate candy all through both days, and I don't eat candy very often.

I need you to take note of something I did right at the beginning of this program, because I think it was important and instrumental in my success. Please notice that I hadn't even started the HCG diet yet and was entering my first binge day. At this point, I actually told everyone around me – not just a few people – that I was doing this. I was shoveling food into the hole in the bottom of my face, and I was telling people around me that it was in order to lose weight. I looked crazy. I was telling people around me – whom I respected, who respected me, whom I considered colleagues – that I was going to lose weight and I was going to be injecting myself with hormones from pregnant women every morning.

Do you see here that there was a huge chance for me to fail? There was a huge chance that I would be humiliated and that, months later, when I saw these people again, they'd poke fun at me, saying, "Remember when you were going to do that diet and you were binge eating?" I had a choice. Once I told them what I was doing, I was either going to see them again and hear, "Remember that?" or see them again and hear, "Oh my God, that worked." It's fitting that I wrote this very paragraph after another work event, which those people attended. All I heard all night was, "Where did the rest of you go?" That's close enough to "Oh my God, that worked," for me.

I think telling them what I was committing to do ended up causing me to work harder toward the end goal, and it played a role in my success. Along the way, it also helped that people knew I was on this diet, because most of them were more likely to help me along by understanding when I couldn't attend events with them where a lot of eating and drinking was going down.

I'm glad I told everyone. I recommend it.

I've known others who have started this plan and who have decided to keep it a secret. They've been embarrassed about the fact that they felt they needed the HCG to succeed, and they also know that others consider this "extreme." I think mainly, though, they're worried about failure. They're worried that if they share what they're doing and it doesn't work out, they will look like they couldn't do it. I think the truth is the other way around.

By sharing this, you have a lot more on the line.
By sharing this, you're less likely to fail.
By not sharing it, you're almost giving yourself a
pass to fail.
You don't want that.

I'll summarize an oft-contested story of Hernán Cortés. Cortés was a Spanish conquistador who was attempting to colonize the Yucatan Peninsula and, with very low chances of his army succeeding, he told them to "burn the ships" on which they sailed in, making retreat impossible. There was only one option – victory!

I challenge you to "burn the ships" by telling everyone you know that you're doing this. Leave yourself no way out! Commit! Like Cortés landing on the shores of Mexico, you must "burn the ships," so that there's no way out of this other than success. Never look back. Tell everyone a new, skinnier, healthier you is on the way, and then fight with every ounce of strength you have to make it happen.

When I sat there getting my vial of HCG from the nutritionist, one thing went through my head again and again was that I was going to need to get the support of my friends and family.

If I didn't tell people I was doing this, my close friends just wouldn't get it. I'd go to restaurants and order strangely: "I'll just have a piece of fish and some asparagus." My friends would have given me an hour and a half of flak about it. I mean, honestly, even after knowing what I was doing, my friends *still* gave me an hour and a half of flak about it, but at least at the end, they'd say, "Hey, seriously – we get it. We understand." And it was that last sentence that made the difference. They helped me through it and even held me accountable in the toughest times. Had I tried to do this without their support, I don't think it would have worked.

You need to tell the people who influence you most that you're doing this, and you need to humbly and sincerely ask for their help.

WEEK ONE: THROWING OUT THE BAD FOOD

PRETTY MUCH ANY MAJOR diet program or weight loss regimen will have you purge your entire kitchen before beginning, and I suggest the same. Atkins.com actually provides a list of things to throw away, as does med-health. net's write-up on the Dr. Oz Ultimate Diet.[60]

As I entered Phase 2 and closed out my "binge phase," I took this step. I threw away all of the food in my entire condo that was not prescribed by my nutritionist for the HCG Phase 2 diet. It's simple.

If it's there, you will probably eat it.

There are going to be times when you are very tempted to eat something that is not on your plan. When this happens, you do not want anything around that you could binge on. I found this out the hard way by leaving some ketchup in the refrigerator. After a week, I was craving sugar so badly that I started putting the ketchup on the saltines that I had for my "starch" servings. I was supposed to eat four of them at a time, only twice a day at most. I felt terrible after "binging" on a full sleeve of saltines and a lot of ketchup. I should have ditched the ketchup from the get-go.

I found the same thing happened one night when I was craving pizza and knew I had some whole wheat tortillas left over from the initial "purge." Guess what? I ate them. Guess what my nutritionist's question was after I gained weight that week: "Where'd you get the tortillas?"

"They were left over in the cabinet."

"Mmmhmm," was her answer.

If there are others in your house who will eat it, this chapter's advice may be tough (but not impossible) to employ. However, if you are living alone or with a very supportive partner who is willing to give up snack foods for a bit while you do this, get rid of the food. Now, your conscience will tell you not to throw food away. You will say things in your head like, "It's wasting food to get rid of this," which it is. If you do live with others, I still think it would be to your advantage (and theirs) to decide together on which foods are okay to get out of the house. You may be surprised about how willing your family is to come to your aid when you've decided to truly commit to this positive change!

You will also say things like, "There are hungry people who need this food," and there are.

I will tell you this. You will either not eat it, or you will eat it. You have two options. One: Throw the food away. Two: Donate the food to a place that will give it to people who need it. *There is no option three, even if your brain seems to think there should be an option.*

Again, like Cortés, you must "burn the ships," leaving any trace of your old life behind, including the food you used to eat!

FEELING DEPRIVED

EVEN WITH MOST OF the bad food thrown out, the first week of Phase 2 was difficult. Following the binge days of Phase 1, I was excited to get started on the actual weight loss portion of the plan. I would wake up each morning, use my countertop Frigidaire grill to cook some chicken and asparagus with various seasonings, and head off to work. At work, I would be careful to drink enough water, eat only exactly what I was supposed to on the plan, and limit my stresses when possible.

At times during Week 1, I got crabby with people. It certainly wasn't easy eating very little. My energy levels were low at times, but I never got to the point where I felt like fainting, which I was worried about after watching an episode of *The Dr. Oz Show* in which a previous HCG user described her experience. At the time, I was fortunate that I was still feeling driven enough to lose the weight that I was able to push the hunger aside. I was still fueled by my initial passion for this goal, and it would carry me through with just enough motivation to last until the weight loss was showing and I became re-inspired. Whenever I got hungry, I would tell myself that hunger was the physical sensation of my belly melting away! It helped.

The best part about Phase 2 for me was that I began to lose weight instantly. On my second binge day, I was at 222.5 pounds. By the end of Week 1, I was at 214 pounds, a full eight and a half pounds down from my max. I hadn't been 214 pounds for a long time, and that felt great!

I was pretty much 10 pounds down after only one week. I still wasn't fitting into my clothes correctly, but I was feeling positive. My mood was one of hope. I was on my way and I felt good. No, I felt *amazing*. Honestly, I was flat-out happy. Let's take a moment to talk about that.

WEEK TWO: ON HAPPINESS AND INITIAL WEIGHT LOSS

"Happiness is the only good. The time to be happy is now. The place to be happy is here. The way to be happy is to make others so." -Robert G. Ingersoll

HERE'S A SECRET.

You don't need to wait to be happy.

Think about happiness. It's what you want, isn't it? We all think that way. *If I could just get to point B, I'd be happy.* What will it really take? Do you know? When you say that to yourself, are you ever really right? Looking back at your life, at the times when you've actually reached the "point B" you were striving for, were you really happy?

I'm pleased to tell you that, for me, happiness came almost right after starting this program. Within days. Here's how it worked for me.

The first time I realized I was losing weight, I got excited. I mean, I was expecting it, but seeing the actual result was invigorating! Then, as I continued to lose day after day,

I realized that it was real. I realized this was sustainable. I realized that this was really, really happening.

When I made the realization that I was able to sustain this rate of weight loss, and that the rate of progress was a reality, I got happy really, really fast.

After about five pounds of weight loss, nobody was noticing my results, but the results were there. I knew it, and I saw that all I had to do was continue my behaviors, and the results would follow. I was *jacked.* Throughout the rest of the process, I was smiling ear to ear. Momentum had started to catch. Every time I felt hungry, I felt great. I felt like that hunger was the feeling of my excess body mass disappearing.

I've found that, for me, happiness in life is much more about the things I look forward to and much less about the things I have. Think about the feeling of elation you get in the weeks before you're about to leave on a big vacation. Get this. Researchers who studied 1,530 Dutch adults found that those planning a vacation were happier than those not going away, yet there was no difference in the happiness of the vacationers and non-vacationers following the vacation![61] This made sense to me. I was happier when I was 10 pounds away from my goal than I was the day I hit it!

For me, happiness has always come from looking *forward* to achieving a goal or from being on the verge of something truly great. Happiness won't be the day I publish this book. Happiness will come for me when I reach the point that I know that publishing this book is about to become a reality.

I've already mentioned Bill Phillips, author of *Body for Life*. In *Body for Life*, Phillips said that people need to focus more on *progress* than results.[62] Phillips argued that if people could get happy about seeing those incremental wins, they'd be a lot more satisfied with life than if they were to spend each day wishing for the end goal. He was right.

When I had lost only 10 pounds, I started to have some fun just shopping for clothes that never would have fit before. I was happy because I could wear pants I hadn't worn in years! I was tucking my shirts in, and I hadn't been able to tuck in my shirts, in recent times anyway. My red belt buckle belly spot went away. My shirts weren't stretched across my chest! Before I started this program, I wouldn't buy a pair of shoes I liked because I felt like I looked bad in them. *Shoes*! Why? I had grown so disappointed with myself that I had "given up," and the thought that went through my head as I looked in the shoe store mirror was, *Dude, you're downright unattractive. Shoes don't matter. Why even spend the money to dress it up?* That was one of my last nights of frustration before I went to the doctor's office.

Within only a couple of weeks, I was waking up elated, every single morning.

Happiness is right around the corner. You just need to focus on progress.

One of the great things about the HCG diet is that you see progress so quickly that you get to experience happiness quickly as well! Within only a week, as you see that progress, you'll realize it's working like nothing has worked for you before, and you'll be smiling ear to ear, waking up happy to run to the scale just like I was. That's exciting! That creates momentum! You're on your way!

When you set out on Phase 1, you may think it will be only one month until you experience happiness from your weight loss, but the truth is, you may be only a week or two away from seeing unbelievable results.

This momentum quickly becomes unstoppable. You'll be amazed at what you keep doing once you start doing it. After you've had three bottles of water, the fourth is easy. After you've lost ten pounds in ten days, the eleventh is a breeze. It will be your expectation to wake up a pound lighter. You won't cheat for a second because you know that you're on a path. If you can carry it just long enough, it will carry you cleanly through the last few weeks! On days when you feel hungry but hold out from eating until bedtime, that happiness will carry you through and put you to sleep before you get that late-night snack. Let progress be your inspiration!

SETBACKS AND ACCOUNTABILITY

BACK TO THE STORY. This is where things got awesome. Too awesome, in fact.

I was doing well and I felt that I had earned the right to give myself a little slack. Here is some background on the night that happened.

Almost by accident, I recently became a part-time professional musician. I have always played guitar and, after college, I took vocal lessons to learn to sing. I put those together and started playing at bars to make a few extra dollars while I tried hard to get by as a first-year stockbroker. At the time, I also thought it would be a good way to meet women, which it is *not*. By the time you're done playing and packing all of your stuff up at 2:00 A.M., any woman who seemed interested in you during your last set has left already with a hunk. Damn hunks.

One of the only perks of being a small-time professional musician is that you get to drink for free. The bar is happy to pay you in beer instead of in American currency, and I am normally happy to receive that form of compensation. As I've mentioned to you, when I have one drink, things are fine, but I'll probably ask for another drink. If you give me another drink, I'll then probably ask for yet another drink.

I guess I should put it this way. Derrick is the one playing the guitar.

When Derrick is stuck behind a microphone for four hours, singing alone to a group of people who aren't even listening because they're focused on their dinner conversations and friends, he just might continue drinking all night.

On an occasion toward the end of Week 2, Derrick did just that.

This brings us to the worst time I cheated on my HCG plan. I had some drinks and I mentally quit on myself that night. I ate some extra food (the aforementioned ketchup on crackers) and I gained some weight. The bad news about this is that I gained some weight and I failed myself. The good news is that this cheating made me feel so bad (both physically and emotionally) that it never happened again to that same extent.

In one morning, I really, truly *did* learn my lesson.

Trust me. You're going to be so pissed off at yourself that you never cheat again.

Honestly, after that night, I really never did cheat nearly as badly again. There were nights where I ate too much or drank a couple of drinks, but there was never another true "cheat night," where I went and binged and blew it. One of those nights was all I needed to decide I was going to see this plan through until I reached my goal.

Though I never had another significant "cheat," I did make some bad decisions along the way.

Here's one for you. I was watching *The Biggest Loser*, which I watched almost constantly as I lost weight, and they presented a tip to make little pizzas using whole wheat tortilla crusts. I thought, *This seems like a great idea. I should try it.* The recipe called for the use of whole grain tortillas as crusts and various normal pizza toppings. I am such a pizza fanatic (as is Derrick) that I assumed this was a great thing to try. It didn't work. When I tried it (I did this a couple of times before I realized it was a mistake), instead of waking up to a pound or two of weight loss, I woke up with a flat line – zero loss, zero gain. Zero pounds of weight gain or loss is fine in one of the maintenance phases, but it's bad in Phase 2!

Later, in Phase 4, I would find out that my body had a particular hate for cheese and that any time I got near cheese, I would gain weight. *As a caveat, Dr. Oz backs this, arguing that cheese contains saturated fats, which are inflammatory, and this is the reason that people tend to put weight on when they eat cheese.*[63]

The important thing about this time for me was that I learned that "cheating" slowed my momentum, no matter what. Even though during those weeks I would average out to a seven-pound-per-week loss, I still didn't like how it impeded my steady losses, so I cut any extras out of the picture.

By the last few weeks of Phase 2, cheating was *done* for me. It just wasn't worth it anymore to cheat, because I knew that if I had even red wine or too many starches or cheese or sugary pizza sauce, it could cause me to plateau for a day, and I hated that more than I hated the "going without."

You might think that after I did all of this the wrong way, that I would tell you not to cheat on HCG. Sure, I'll say that. I'll also say that it's silly to think you won't, because I believe that you will. I mean, you've spent your whole life developing your habits, why would either of us believe you'd make a change and start behaving perfectly now? We shouldn't, so we don't.

Here's the most important thing I can tell you about cheating while on your plan. It doesn't mean anything. So you screwed up. Fine. So you had a lapse in judgment. Fine. Keep going, at all costs.
Stay the course.
Stay the course.
Stay the course.
Stay the course.

I can tell you that when I cheated and had some weight gain, I felt guilt immediately the next morning. I would wake up and feel terrible. I would think, *Why did I do that?* Worse, a fear deep inside of me would whisper in my ear that this just might be that "turning point" where I start to gain weight and I never go back to my weight loss. I would think of each cheat instance as some monumental event that would lead to my future obesity. I was wrong when I was thinking that way.

When you eat a piece of cake, it is not a turning point. It is simply a piece of cake. When you cheat on the plan, it does not need to be a turning point. It's one cheat. It's one lapse in judgment. It's very, very fixable. Look at it that way. Don't give it significance it doesn't deserve.

Wake up the next day, grab yourself some coffee, and within 45 minutes you'll be back on your plan, doing just fine. Nutritionist Daphne Sashin says, "Don't try to make up for the extra calories by skipping meals the next day. That just leaves you hungry."[64] Say to yourself, *it's going to be just fine*. Again, ***it's going to be just fine!*** Just keep thinking that and keep progressing forward. Do not let a cheat event ruin your momentum. It absolutely can, *if you let it*, but it doesn't have to, because you can control it. A lapse in judgment is only a lapse in judgment, not some monumental milestone in your life. You're bigger than that. It was what it was. Give yourself a break, hit the damn gas pedal, and get back on the road.

I love the movie *Vanilla Sky*. There's just something so powerful about it. My favorite quote from the movie is this: "Every passing minute is another chance to turn it all around." Think about that. Say it to yourself.

There are no "streaks." People create those, but they don't exist on their own.

Sure, the best way to predict someone's behavior today is to look at what he or she did yesterday. People tend to repeat the same behaviors.

However.

Remember that with knowledge and preparation, you still have the ability to choose what you will do in any given minute. You can choose to let your patterns dictate your life or you can choose to prepare yourself to change those patterns. When you fall back into an old habit, you can think through it before the cause of the consequence occurs and push forward into the new habit you want to pursue. When your old habits guide you and cause you to lapse, fine, just make sure you turn back toward the light and keep walking as soon as you can. Keep trying. Keep going. Don't give up. Forgive yourself for lapses in judgment. Move on. Look back, chuckle because you screwed up, and realize that whether that screw-up has any bearing on your future is completely up to you, in this moment. It doesn't have to. Keep going, at all costs. Remember *Vanilla Sky*: *"Every passing minute is another chance to turn it all around."*

My nutritionist is a Godsend. I'm so thankful to have her guidance and advice. One of the best things I could have done was to go to my doctor and ask for help. My nutritionist was that help. Every week I would meet with her on or around Tuesday morning. I'd go there, weigh in, and tell her about what I'd done that week. Most weeks I'd lose about five to seven pounds, so she'd be happy with me. Having said that, when she really helped was when she was *not* happy with me.

When I went in and told my nutritionist about the binge night I had while playing guitar at the bar, followed by a night where I had taken down some wine at a gala, she did something I'll always be thankful for. She asked me, "What's with the alcohol?"

She (very intentionally) didn't say, "Oh, that's fine, everyone does that." She didn't say, "We all have a drink now and then." She said, "What's with the alcohol?"

Trust me when I tell you that my nutritionist was coming from a very good, sincere place in doing what she did, which was looking at me like she was looking at an addict. She took some time to question me about why I couldn't control myself for even a few months to make a better life and a better future for myself. In that moment I thought, *There is no way on earth I am going to let someone look at me like I'm an out-of-control addict. I'm stronger than that, and I'm going to fix this.*

After that point, I gave up the alcohol until my weight loss goal was met.

Because my nutritionist had been there to hold me accountable, I was able to finish strong. Had I not gone in to see her that day, I would have probably cheated again. Having her support (but, more importantly, her honestly and her ability to directly challenge my behavior) made me better. I'm grateful for that.

Psychology Today says, "A crucial ingredient in any successful weight loss or maintenance program is accountability. In fact, it's nearly impossible to maintain your weight loss without a strong system of accountability. It's not enough to be accountable to oneself, as it becomes too easy to rationalize poor decisions. When accountable, giving inadequate excuses to someone who is holding your feet to the fire becomes much more difficult."[65]

I was lucky to have my nutritionist to hold me accountable. No, I wasn't just lucky. I made the decision to compensate a professional to hold me accountable, and that made all the difference.

So, all-in-all, I got through a tough time, I forgave myself, and I got right back onto schedule after being held accountable by my nutritionist.

It never ceases to amaze me when I see people shopping around online to find the lowest price possible for HCG. The value of a nutritionist who will make sure you get quality HCG, and who will monitor your progress and hold you accountable, *far* outweighs the small amount of money that can be saved by shopping for HCG from a shady source. How much would you pay to really, truly lose the amount of weight you want to? $300? $500? $1,000? More? That being the case, why would you look to save money by avoiding the one thing that helps more than any other – your healthcare team? I think that if you're still in the mindset where you're not ready to take this seriously enough to consult a professional, but you're shopping online for hormones, you're not ready. You're still in a mindset of looking for shortcuts, and not in one where you're ready to make a lasting change and pay your dues. Fast weight loss and lasting change are possible, but the process feels nothing like a shortcut, and it's going to take a mental and financial commitment.

I will tell you this about what I believe you should do: find a nutritionist who is close to work or home and make yourself show up to every single appointment. Even if you cheated, get in there and confess! When you walk out, whether you were scolded or praised, you'll feel better about the upcoming week. At times, if you cheat, you'll be tempted to cancel or skip your weekly visit. Don't do that. Go in. Take the reprimand, then put your chin up, take the advice you get, and move on. Remember, this is someone you pay to hold you accountable. Confide in her. Tell her the truth. Tell her exactly what you did so she can yell at you and it can be behind you. Don't hold back. This is someone who will tell you the truth – not like your spouse who doesn't want to see you in pain, and might say, "It's okay to have a little ice cream."

On this note, remember that your spouse or partner is not paid to get you skinny and tell you the truth and for that reason might actually be a deterrent to your good behavior. Your spouse is not the one who you should listen to about weight loss. Your nutritionist and doctor are! Also know that by staying strong, you might influence your spouse to follow along in your path. Research published in the *International Journal of Obesity* shows that the reach of behavioral weight loss treatment can extend to a spouse![66]

As a final note in this chapter, I'll recommend that you select a nutritionist, like I did, who doesn't mind you emailing him or her frequently. You need to have an accountability partner here, and that means you need someone who is responsive, who cares about you, and who sees his or her job as getting you to the finish line. That means off-hours communication is sometimes necessary. When you're interviewing nutritionists, ask if they're willing to be that "hands-on." If he or she is not, find someone who is. There are so many "HCG dealers" out there who just want to sell you the hormones and take their cut of the cash. The hormone, in my experience, is the smallest element that affects change here, and your healthcare professionals are a bigger element of the change. Make sure to select your partner in this, using your highest level of scrutiny.

WEEK THREE: VACATION, PEOPLE NOTICING, AND NEW CLOTHES

WEEK 3 OF PHASE 2 was interesting for me, because it involved a previously-planned vacation. All in all, it was a great trip. I continued to lose weight throughout the trip, and had a blast.

I think there were three things that made this vacation a "weight loss success."

First, my preparation was key. Throughout the vacation, I was able to eat the proteins, vegetables, and fruits that I needed, because I'd packed enough to eat for the whole trip, just in case. My HCG was on ice, and I was able to find an ice machine to stock the cooler, making sure the HCG didn't get too warm.

The second factor in my success on vacation was that there were so many great restaurants in the area to choose from. Now, upscale restaurants were much more affordable because I wasn't ordering appetizers, drinks, side items, or desserts! I was able to get away with going to some fancier places while not spending so much money because the only cost was for a small entrée and a vegetable. I looked forward to meals at great restaurants where I knew the food would be delicious, even though it would be minimalist eating for me! I had been eating my own cooking up until this point, and it was just great to get to a couple of restaurants where I could have a piece of fish that was prepared perfectly by a chef, along with some steamed vegetables that somebody made with the kind of skill I just don't have. I loved every bite of my food that weekend.

The third reason the vacation went as well as it did was that I was able to avoid alcohol. If you're like me, you like to enjoy a few drinks when you're on a vacation, and that can be problematic if you're working on losing weight. Research published in the *American Journal of Clinical Nutrition* shows that eliminating alcohol consumption is key in weight loss as alcohol limits the body's ability to burn fat. According to the authors, the alcohol calories you consume aren't stored, but instead, they're converted to acetate, a type of fuel that the body burns quickly. As a result, you burn off your alcohol calories before you burn the fat you are trying to eliminate by increasing your exercise and cutting back on your food intake.[67] Most importantly, the advice I received from my nutritionist was not to drink, and so I wasn't drinking at all at this point.

So often, we make the next things we look forward to in life about meals and about "treats." Some look forward to that cigarette break. Some look forward to that big meal they're going to have. So, my advice to myself (which worked) was, *Let's change that.* Let's instead look forward to an amazing small steak at a nice restaurant. Let's look forward to the best small plate of vegetables we've ever had. Let's look forward to seeing how a world-class chef can prepare the meals we've been trying to cook on our own at home. Let's look forward to a nice massage and a stroll on the beach at a great resort. When I started looking forward to these things instead of just an unhealthy meal or even a drink, I found myself even happier than I'd been in the past, because I felt much better physically than I did after having a huge meal.

In summary, the trip was a success, and I experienced even more weight loss while we were traveling. I even did a little shopping for clothes while I was in Coronado, because I realized I could fit into a few things I wouldn't have been able to before! Being straight-forward with you, I didn't buy anything because it was all so expensive. Regardless, trying things on was more fun than it used to be.

Week 3 was actually the week of my transformation when people began to notice my progress. Three people I worked with during this week actually commented that I was looking slimmer and asked what I was doing. It was working! Between the productive and relaxing vacation and the compliments I was getting, this was a fantastic week, and it helped me to build momentum.

WHAT TO LOOK FORWARD TO

I WANT TO TAKE a moment to go a bit deeper on this topic of "looking forward" to things. I think we all look forward to things, and that's often what helps us get through the day.

When you dedicate yourself to a weight loss plan, you start to realize, almost immediately, that you don't have many (if any) of the same things to look forward to that you used to. You will realize that you need to start looking forward to new things, and once you make that conversion happen in your mind, life gets a lot better!

As part of the "know thyself" strategy, I suggest that right now, whatever you're doing and wherever you are, you take a personal inventory of those things you look forward to. What is it that you're looking forward to tonight? Write it down. Does it revolve around food? Does it revolve around drinks? The more you can identify even the tiniest things that you're looking forward to and then ensure that those things are healthy and compliant with the program that you've chosen to follow, the better your mood will become.

For me, as I mentioned, I started to look forward to great meals instead of looking forward to big meals. I started

looking forward to a new flavor of coffee instead of looking
forward to a breakfast buffet. I started looking forward to
getting home and doing some grilling while watching *The
Biggest Loser*, instead of heading out to a restaurant. I got to
know my new life, and I got to like my new life. These new
habits, combined with my progress, made me a happier guy
all around, and those habits have stuck with me since the
transformation occurred.

So, what's on your list? Write it down and, if you need
to, make some changes! Here are some of my favorite things
that I still, to this day, look forward to:

- A great cup of coffee, even if it's decaf at night

- An ice cold San Pellegrino sparkling water (this re-
placed Monster and Rockstar energy drinks for me!)

- A big omelet in the morning, with a little sausage and a
lot of peppers (no cheese!)

- Some time to just unwind while cooking my dinner
and packing up the next day's food

- Waking up early and getting a chance to relax and journal before the day begins

- Just spending time with my loved ones and pets

- Just waking up and realizing I get to be thin and healthy
today!

- A nice dinner with a perfectly cooked piece of fish at a great restaurant with a delectable veggie I've never tasted before, and maybe a glass of cabernet (I'm now in Phase 4 so I get to do that sometimes!)

Whatever it is that you choose to look forward to, it's important that you take this time to be deliberate about changing your old thought patterns and replacing them with new ones.

WEEK FOUR: FINDING DISCIPLINE

WEEK 4 WAS A fun week for me, because others at work started to ask what I'd changed. It was hilarious when someone actually asked me if my hair was getting longer (when the truth was my cheeks were just getting smaller!). I was down another belt notch, and I was starting to fit into my clothes even better.

The toughest part about Week 4 was that it occurred between Thanksgiving and Christmas, and that meant a work holiday party with all sorts of bad influences.

Our organization puts on a great party every year where everyone gets dressed up and heads to an upscale venue. It's a really neat event, and I always like to attend, but this year I dreaded having to be surrounded by temptation! This year, the party was stocked with the most delicious looking food, including mini sliders and a hot dog bar. I was surrounded by foods I could not eat and wanted to eat badly. It was tough also, because the drinks were flowing freely and everyone there was having a great time, grabbing drinks and dancing and such. I knew it was going to be a tough night of temptation, and it was. I also felt very prepared for it, because I had deliberately thought it through.

The way I got through this was as follows. First, my plan was to work as *hard* as I could to "make an appearance," by seeing as many people as I could very quickly, before getting the heck out of there, away from the temptation! I had the pleasure but temptation/disadvantage of accompanying my girlfriend, who was seeing friends she almost never gets to see and was intent on staying and talking to people. What she didn't realize was that I was so tempted by that food and those drinks that I needed to leave! Worse, she was eating the stuff! Because she was healthy, she was able to pack in appetizers like the LA Beast (a competitive eater who just might be my hero[68]). The problem was that she didn't realize that I was an addict and that I was surrounded by the things I was addicted to. It was terrible. I literally had to do something rude and walk in front of her on the way out of the place, just to get her to follow me, because she wanted to stay and chat with people. I hated having to do that, and I did feel bad about it, but, honestly, it exemplifies what's needed when you want to make a change like this.

Sometimes (and this time is one of those times), you need to do things for you, so that you can be successful in this weight loss phase. While you're trying to change your habits, as rude as it may be, you're going to need to get yourself out of situations where you know you're going to do the wrong thing. You can have the food and the drinks later, but for now, it's critical that you don't. So, you need to be very, very clear with the people you're closest to that you're making this your first priority and that, even though it's the holiday party, you're leaving early!

The week following the party, I developed a sense of extreme discipline, due to my progress, paired with the on-coming end to the weight loss and accomplishment of my goal.

My motto became (and often still is):
"Wake up proud."

My whole thought was focused on being proud of who I was when I woke up. Each night of sleep was like a reset for me. It was an end to the prior day, closing out a day of discipline, and I'd wake up lighter, excited to face the next day and drop another pound.

The best part about Week 4 was that I was close to the end, and even though I wasn't really getting a lot of com-pliments on my weight loss just yet, I knew I was chang-ing and I knew I was close to being seen as having made a massive transformation. The kind of discipline that got me to leave that party early was the discipline that carried me through a very strong final week, to my final weight, seven pounds lower. Those final seven pounds made all the dif-ference, and I was literally a different person by the end.

WEEK FIVE: FUN THINGS TO TELL PEOPLE ABOUT HOW YOU LOST WEIGHT

WE'VE COME TO THE point where I'm about to make a massive transformation, and people are going to start to notice. When you get here yourself, it's time to have a little fun. I tried to think of as many ways as possible to tell people what the heck had happened. In this final week, people were approaching me left and right and asking me what I did! My transformation was going well enough that people were even asking me if my weight loss was intentional. I think they saw such a dramatic change that *seemed* positive, but was almost unbelievable due to its rapid pace, so they were even worried to ask me about it! I didn't look sickly or anything – I was looking more energetic and healthy – I think it's just not often you see someone shrink that quickly.

So, as a reward for coming this far with me on the journey, I'll share with you some of the things I told people when they asked what was going on with me. I really did use each of these at least once, if not more.

"My Jillian Michaels tape got stuck in my VCR. It's all I can watch, and once it's on, I can't stop doing the exercises."

"I'm wearing Spanx."

"I got liposuction."

"Six-Minute Abs."

"I became a Zumba instructor."

"I'm wearing a wrestling singlet under my clothes. It feels good." Then, I'd get into a wrestling stance sometimes.

And my favorite…

"I wake up every morning and inject myself with pregnant lady hormones while eating 500 calories per day."

The last one – and the most unbelievable of the whole lot – is the only one that's true. Well, except for the Spanx, but that's not an everyday thing.

THE FINAL STRETCH AND REWARDING MYSELF

WEEK 5 WAS A week of *absolute discipline*. Every day I ate perfectly. My journal shows I literally lost one and a half pounds the first day, gained a half-pound the next, lost two and a half the next, lost another half the next, then another full pound the next. It was a great week of discipline, and I decided with my nutritionist that I was at the end of my Phase 2.

We had done it. We really, really had done it.

We had a good discussion and decided to switch over to maintenance phase. I can't tell you how good it felt to close out those last few days, just walking around being a new "me." Just taking a stroll felt good! Just getting out of bed and putting on a shirt I never could have worn before felt good! Life was new and exciting. I was invigorated! Even better, it was time to reward myself.

This is when I would like to clue you in on something I did along the way to keep me motivated the whole way through this program. I've always tried to avoid conspicuous consumption, and this next part may sound a bit excessive, but I'm really spilling my guts here and I need to tell the whole story and the truth, so here goes.

Since I was a young guy in the working world, I had always wanted a nice watch. I never bought one for a host of reasons, including the fact that I thought it was just wasteful, and that the watch I always wanted was pricey and it just didn't seem right to spend money on it. I'm a huge fan of Dave Ramsey and Suze Orman, and as someone who worked as a Financial Advisor, and even did a fair share of writing on personal finance, I just always knew it wasn't a smart move. Honestly, I still don't think it's a smart move!

It's not important that I tell you what kind of watch it is – it's just one I really liked a lot. When I started at my job in finance, one of the really successful brokers I worked with had this watch, and I just loved the look of it. When I found out how much it cost him, I realized it was totally out of my price range, and I quickly gave up the thought of picking one up.

Funny enough, at my next job, when people were promoted, they would get this exact same watch as a gift. This was such a neat thing, but I was on a different career path from the people who would be promoted into those positions. No matter what I did or what level I was promoted to, nobody was giving me a watch anytime soon (a.k.a. never). I also couldn't buy one on my own because, frankly, at the time I again just didn't have the money for it. If I *had* the money for it, I would have done something more productive with it, like put it away in savings!

For a long time now I've been very thrifty and have finally put enough money away that I think Suze Orman or Dave Ramsey might not yell at me for spending a little of it.

I got to a point where I could finally buy the watch without breaking the bank. I wanted to do it, but I felt like I needed a reason to! I mean, I'd wanted this thing for about 10 years at this point, and there was no way I was going to just go out and swipe a card and buy it!

Self-reflecting, I'm sure I learned this kind of behavior from my father. When I was young and I really wanted a certain toy, my dad would make me wait for it. He wanted me to learn the value of hard work and didn't want me to think I could just have anything I wanted. I remember back as far as age six, when I wanted nothing more than this AM/FM portable radio (this was the era of the Sony Walkman). I wasn't old enough to do almost anything other than go to school and eat my lunch. So, my dad simply made me wait for it. After weeks of waiting until a specific date, he finally got it for me. It was the coolest thing in the world – I remember listening to it every night for years!

Later, my dad did the same thing but made it even more difficult. I wanted a toy that was expensive, and all of my friends had it. The toy came in pieces, and instead of just buying all six for me, he set up a series of challenges that I had to accomplish to get each piece. I was on the swim team, and he made me tread water for six minutes before I could get the first piece. I had to swim a certain number of consecutive laps to get the second. Each challenge made me stretch myself to accomplish something I didn't think I could achieve. By the time I got that toy, I had worked *hard* for it.

I can think of many examples of my father doing this. One time, I wanted to visit New York City because I was obsessed with the tall buildings. I had an aunt that lived on Long Island, and my dad said we could take a road trip to visit, but first I needed to write a report on all of the tall buildings we'd see, and even create graphics so that we could see them side-by-side. The World Trade Center was always my favorite, and when we finally got there and went up to the observation deck, I was elated. The victory wasn't just because of the obsession – it was because of the hard work I did to get an understanding of the buildings we were going up in.

I was very fortunate to have parents that instilled me with that kind of work ethic, and I sometimes take for granted the fact that I'm unable to let myself do anything without setting goals first. I often need to make myself re-member, *that came from someplace!* I'll be forever grateful for it.

So, as it was with my childhood, it became with my adulthood. It's funny – you can point to anything of value that I own and ask me the question, *What did you make your-self do before you bought it,* and I'll have an answer for you.

In this case, I decided that if I could reach a specific weight (about 30 pounds lighter), I would let myself get the watch. I realized that if I made the purchase about this goal, I'd be very, very proud to wear that watch.

It wasn't just about wearing a piece of jewelry, it was about being proud of an accomplishment and changing my life.

I wrote my goal on my wall chart and I moved forward.

I actually filed the thought of actually accomplishing this goal in the back of my head – I didn't actually think I'd get *that* far. I was dead set on doing it, but I also knew that it was a stretch, and I actually assumed somewhere deep inside that I probably would fall short of the actual watch-related goal.

However, during Week 5, and somewhat to my own disbelief, I realized this thing was actually within reach. I realized I was going to achieve my goal, and because of my recent discipline, I also realized I could time to the very day when I would hit it! I took the plunge, and ordered the watch so that it would arrive the very *day* that I got to my goal weight. It's on my wrist as I type this chapter, and honestly, I feel great about it. To you, this may sound materialistic, and maybe you're right.

Here's what I think though. I think sometimes people want material things for the wrong reasons, and sometimes they want things because they really will enjoy them. I'd wanted this thing for 10 years, and even though it was just a "thing," I made it about a goal and I made it mean something to me. I wasn't putting myself in financial jeopardy by buying it, and every single day it's a reminder to me of the pain that I went through and the discipline I needed to have to make this transformation happen. I got myself to 30 pounds lighter, and I get to wear a reminder of that every day. I think it's pretty neat. I've gone a step further and actually had my goal weight etched into the case of the watch, so it's always there to remind me what I went through to get where I am.

So, why did I explain all this? I explained it because I think that rewarding yourself for accomplishing this goal is important. I think that you should think of a lot of ways to really celebrate achieving this goal. I want you to envision those rewards, every single day when you get out of bed, and all day through the day as you make sacrifices and eat the right foods! What are you going to do to reward yourself? Think about it long and hard and write it down! Later in the book, we'll talk more about using a wall chart and visualization to keep yourself thinking about your bright future. For now, just pick one big reward and get it burned into your mind! I advise you to make it something that will last forever. For women, a handbag (though it might be fun for now) may be a little short-term. Think big! Is it a locket? Is it a trip you visit to a place you've always dreamed of going, with pictures you can keep from the trip? Is it an etched stone in your garden? A piece of artwork or family photo? Whatever it is, it should be something that's always there to remind you of this journey, and to help hold you accountable to not going back to the old habits! Is it a tattoo? I don't know you well, but I bet it's a tattoo. Based on the way you've been reading so far and how this whole interaction is going, I see a tattoo in your skinny future.

"MAKEOVER WEEK"

IF YOU'VE EVER WATCHED *The Biggest Loser,* you've seen "makeover week." This is a week that happens every season where they take the contestants, who are now much skinnier than they were when they started, out on the town for a full makeover with famous stylists and clothing designers. The contestants get haircuts, beard trims, makeup – the works. By the end, you don't even recognize them. I suggest that you look forward to doing the same. Just like they do on the show, I think you should let your hair and beard (for guys) grow out until you get to the end of Phase 2. Let stuff get baggy. Delay the shopping! Then, when you're 30 pounds down or even 40 pounds down, hit the stores and treat yourself to stuff you never could have worn before.

One of the things I did once I lost the weight at the end of Phase 2 was head out and buy a ton of clothes. I mean, I got new sweaters, shoes, jackets, even socks. I actually got lots of neat, colorful socks. If you remember just a few chapters back, I went out to buy shoes before I started my transformation and wouldn't even buy those because I didn't care enough about myself to invest a few bucks to make a difference. Man, how things had changed! It felt great to be able to fit into clothes I never could have worn before!

I bought everything but a belt, because I still enjoyed wearing the belt that I was using to measure my progress. In fact, "enjoyed" is probably an understatement – I was more obsessed with using it to make sure I didn't gain the weight back. To this day, if I'm having a day where I feel like I've cheated too much, I throw that belt back on just to get a quick reality-check. Many times at this point in the journey, which was right between Phase 2 and Phase 3, I'd actually wake up in the morning scared that I was gaining weight back. The belt helped me to ground myself during those times. I'll talk more about that in the next chapter.

I'll go even further and recommend that you get some form-fitting clothing that you never, ever could have worn had you not gone through this process. My favorite items purchased were a couple of form-fitting fleece hoodies that weren't too tight but would have been like shrink-wrap had I worn them before the program. I now wear them, and it just reminds me (and others) that I'm tiny compared to the size I used to be. I love it! I think it's a great mental checkmark and sense of accomplishment that goes along with this transformation. When you come in to work or wherever you are after your own personal makeover week, people will say, "Wow – you look amazing."

Do your hair! (I shaved mine!) Do your makeup (I didn't do this because I'm a guy, but you do what you want – don't hold back!)

To sum it up, I think you should give yourself a make-over week – a full makeover week. Head to a spa, too, if you get a chance. Treat yourself! Enjoy it! You've been through a major challenge, and you're a whole lot better off! This is when people will say, "Holy cow, you're disappearing!" You'll look forward to this week through your entire transformation, and it will be a well-deserved indulgence.

If you want to have some extra fun with this, I'd recommend taking before and after pictures. Take the before pics at the very beginning of your program during your binge days. I took before and after pictures thinking I wouldn't use them much, but I'm so happy I did it. Even though I'm embarrassed to print them in this book, I show them to everyone who asks to see them in person. There was a very dramatic shift in my physique between the time before and the time after this plan. At the beginning, I had a huge, evident "gut." At the end, it was completely gone, along with half of my face, and I looked like a different person!

Finally, it may be a neat bonus for you to find some old clothes before you start your program that you can barely squeeze into. Keep them in a special spot so you can find them easily. Try them on every couple of weeks. You'll be amazed at the changes that occur quickly in Phase 2, and you'll get recharged when you feel the momentum from this. It's possible that by makeover week, they'll fit you perfectly!

THE PHASE 2 TO PHASE 3 TRANSITION: HORMONAL CRAZINESS

THE TRANSITION FROM PHASE 2 to Phase 3 is probably one of the scariest parts of the entire HCG diet plan, because it's where you're done losing the weight, you're nervous about gaining it all back, and you need to increase your caloric intake dramatically so that you reengage your metabolism, while maintaining your last injection weight, or "LIW." It can be a stressful time because of the worry and anxiety that go along with this increased calorie load. The good news is it doesn't have to be stressful if you really trust the plan!

Having said this, I did get stressed – very stressed – as I went through this, and I need to warn you about a very rough day that I had with the transition from Phase 2 to Phase 3. I hope this doesn't happen to you the way it happened to me, but if it does, you'll have this to prepare you for it!

For me, there was one particular day between Phase 2 and Phase 3 that was really hard to get through. On my third day following the completion of my injections, I felt very depressed, which is not like me. I wrote in my journal, "Experienced symptoms of depression today. Felt like an anorexic because I got so worried that my weight had increased." I remember this day vividly. It was a Saturday, and I was very worried that my weight had increased, because I'd had some drinks and some cheese the night before. (I would later find that cheese is the one food that makes me retain weight like no other food out there – I eat even a little cheese and I'm retaining weight for days.)

I got all worried because I was supposed to increase my caloric intake to begin to establish my new set point and increase my metabolism, yet I was already up three pounds from my "LIW." So, I did a "correction day" (later, we'll talk about "steak days" which are used to correct your weight when you gain too much) and brought my weight back down. The problem was, all through the day I felt depressed. I was up in my head bouncing thoughts around so vividly that I couldn't believe it. I went to see a movie that I had really been looking forward to, and I couldn't concentrate, even for a minute. I ended up going in to the office to do some work just to get my mind off of things. It was a really hard day! Now, the good thing is that as I got to the office I realized what was happening. I was being hormonal!

Don't forget, my friend, that HCG is a hormone, and you've been *injecting* yourself with it for weeks now – more than a month, every day. When you cut that out, you can't expect that things are just going to stay perfectly the same up in your head! I had some pregnant friends at the time who were often emotional, and I ran into one of them that day. I was thinking, "Man, this pregnant lady seems emotional," and then I thought, "I'm acting like a pregnant lady today." I immediately realized that I had been injecting pregnant lady hormones into my belly for a month and had recently gone cold turkey.

I did some reading, spoke with my nutritionist, and found that it is normal to experience some emotional swings during this period. I found that my chemistry was screwing with me. It wasn't nearly as bad the next day and went away completely about two days later. It was only one full day that I really felt the full effect of the emotional swings.

My advice to you here is to talk with your doctor and nutritionist to make sure you're ready for it. I was able to laugh it off when it hit me, even though it was tough to deal with in the moment. I recognized that it wasn't "me," thinking these thoughts, but it was a hormonal imbalance, and that I just needed to get through it by maintaining the self-realization that I was going through a hormonal transition, and that it would pass.

If you're like I was, there will be a very rational fear that you carry with you for a bit at this point, that you're going to gain the weight back, but I'll say this: After only about a month of maintenance, I realized that I was at a new "set point" for my body weight, and I felt indestructible. As I've said many times before, the key here is to stick to the plan given to you by your doctor and nutritionist. This is the way through the tough times!

MAKING A MENU FOR PHASE 3

ONE THING THAT INSTANTLY became a pain when I entered Phase 3 was the fact that I had to eat a *lot* more calories, but it all needed to be healthy. Preparation for Phase 2 was easy. I had to eat so little that it was very easy to prepare a couple of tiny pieces of fish, chicken, or steak and a couple of veggies. In Phase 2, I could have kept my entire day's food in my pockets (if I had cargo pants) or maybe a fanny pack.

Phase 3 required a lot more cooking and a lot more transportation of food. Thank goodness I'd gotten used to cooking in Phase 2, because without that transition stage, I could have never had the knowledge or stamina to cook what I needed for Phase 3.

I struggled at first to do this, and then I found a great way of doing it that I'll share with you here.

Previously, to track the foods I needed to eat in Phase 2, I was using a list from my nutritionist that was based on "servings per day." I had transferred this list into an iPhone app called Clear, which I'll explain in more detail later in this book. For now, know that I had been tracking my meals using a checklist of actual servings (think one protein, one vegetable, one fruit).

The thing that helped me most in this transition was changing over to a menu of meals instead of the checklist of servings.

Here's how to do it.

Get out a notecard and write down a whole day of eating that includes three to five meals and possibly some snacks – however you want to set it up, in line with your nutritionist's advice. This time, you're going to group your servings into meals. So, instead of thinking *I have to have two servings of protein and two servings of vegetables this morning,* you'll just think, *I'm going to have an omelet this morning. That omelet will contain two servings of protein (four to six eggs) and two servings of vegetables (half a pepper, half an onion, half a tomato, and some mushrooms).* You'll also get one healthy oil serving into that omelet by using a healthy oil to cook it with. By adding a half grapefruit, you can cover a fruit serving. Now, things are a lot easier to see, and to check off. Your omelet and grapefruit just got you through two proteins, two vegetables, an oil, and a fruit for the morning!

Visually, the note card consisted of a simple, 4" by 6" ruled card, with one line on it representing each meal of the day. Line one read, "Breakfast – one omelet (4 – 6 eggs, 2 whole veg, oil) + ½ grapefruit." Line two read, "Snack – yogurt with berries." The card helped me to group all of these servings together into easy-to-envision meals. Each meal took up one line on the card.

I've mentioned this, and I'll mention it again, omelets are a great way for people who don't usually eat big, whole servings of vegetables to get some good veggies into their systems. I use them a lot for this! Plus, it turns out that eating eggs has an added bonus! Tim Ferris, author of *The 4 Hour Body: An Uncommon Guide To Rapid Fat Loss, Incredible Sex, And Becoming Superhuman,* encourages readers to eat eggs within 30 minutes of waking up for maximum weight loss.[69]

Omelets can even provide meals for a full day. If I'm in a rush, I might even make a *giant* omelet that can be broken up into multiple servings, so that if I put it in a big storage container and eat it all day at work, it takes care of all of my protein and veggies for the day.

I've also done this with stuffed peppers, a great tip I got from *The Biggest Loser.* I'll cut a pepper in half, and stuff it with very low-fat ground beef, turkey, or chicken, and add a mix of chopped vegetables to the meat, including peppers, onions, mushrooms, and tomatoes. It's a very tasty way to get more vegetables into your system.

As you get used to writing down meals instead of servings, you'll develop a notecard that includes your menu for the whole day. The notecard will be very simple to follow. It will have four to five meals listed on it, that will all be simple to prepare and get through.

A second pain point during the transition to Phase 3 for me was that I needed to carry so much food around with me all day. I found, at first, that I was carrying a massive bag back and forth to work, and it was taking me forever each morning to pack the bag with healthy foods.

Remember, now that you're on Phase 3, you want to start developing systems that you can use for the rest of your life. If you find that you're carrying a massive bag of food everywhere you go and that it's not something that you can sustain for good, you're still in "diet" mode and haven't made good, healthy habits that fit into your life yet.

The way to make lasting change is to make changes that are sustainable and become habits.

If you're doing something now that you can't see your-self doing for good, you need to find a better way.

My better way came through the realization that I could store a lot of food in my office. The foods I was eating through the week included breadsticks (which I could bring an entire box of and leave at my desk), olives (which can sit out forever), apples, and pistachios. This significantly lightened the daily load. Then I found that I could make Monday my big "carry day," and I'd use that day to bring yogurt, berries, and cottage cheese. I also stored tons of bottled water at work under my desk, so I didn't need to lug that around, either. The only thing I needed to carry in and out for the rest of the week were my main meals like a salad for lunch, or maybe my lettuce wraps or an omelet. This made it so that I only needed my laptop bag and one small bag for my day's food. By taking the time to plan this way and making sure I was prepared over the weekend for my Monday morning transport, I was able to create a sus-tainable system that's now easy to carry through the rest of my life. Without those sustainable systems, it just wouldn't work for me.

At this point in the journey, I also began to branch out a bit and look for new recipes. I realized that if I was go-ing to sustain this behavior for life, I'd need to add some variety. There are many, many books that exist that are full of recipes that are compliant with the HCG protocol, so I won't go into depth here. I'll just say two things about finding recipes that meet your needs.

First, Pinterest is a great place to find recipes and wonderful foods that you can modify to accommodate the plan that your nutritionist has advised.

Second, Pinterest is a great place to look at a bunch of food that will make you hungry!

Don't look for recipes on Pinterest late at night! All that tasty food will make you go nuts! Do it when you're feeling good and full and satisfied, or at a time of day when you're least likely to binge (for me that was in the early morning).

I was up late one night looking at deviled egg recipes on Pinterest. Until that point I had been sitting there feeling great about my day. After about five recipes, I was craving deviled eggs like never before. Big surprise, right? You'll laugh at me, but it wasn't funny at the time: I ended up binging on mustard and saltines.

I didn't gain a lot because of my binge, but I realize now that late-night in bed is not the place to stare at images of food and read about how to prepare it. Save that for a time you're in more control.

PHASE 3: EXERCISE – TAKING THE NEW BODY FOR A SPIN

ONE OF THE BEST things I got to do once I was comfortably into Phase 3 was to begin exercising again. Before my weight loss, when I had tried to exercise to lose weight, I was sluggish and, of course, heavy. After losing 30 pounds, I went running and I felt like I was flying! I was able to run much farther and faster than I'd run in years. Back before I'd gained weight, I would train for mountain climbs. It had been since then (about five years now) that I'd been overweight to the extent that I couldn't train like I used to. This time, I was even lighter than I'd been back when I was climbing mountains, and I was able to really crank while I was out there. It was exciting to be exercising again and doing so in a much more leisurely, yet powerful way! The weight loss enabled me to have a body that would truly take me to new heights, and it was exciting. It was after just one training run in the morning that I decided I'd do a half marathon in just a few weeks!

Though I didn't have enough time to really train hard for the half-marathon without causing injury, I ended up building up my endurance enough within just a couple of weeks that I was able to run/walk the event and complete it in a reasonable time, within close range of my last half-marathon time from years prior. As I write this book, I'm training for another half-marathon and plan to complete a full marathon later in the year. I owe the ability to train this hard without injury to my weight loss.

I include this because I want critics of these types of plans to understand that even though there is sometimes a cessation of exercise during Phase 2, those who think that they must exercise in order to lose weight are neglecting that it's possible to take a short break from the workouts to focus on shrinking and to come back even stronger. If your healthcare professionals advise that you follow a plan like this, I'd take that advice, because it certainly worked well for me.

"STEAK DAYS" IN PHASE 3

"Have patience with all things, but chiefly have patience with yourself. Do not lose courage in considering your own imperfections but instantly set about remedying them— every day begin the task anew." —Saint Francis de Sales

ONE OF THE TOOLS that can be used to maintain your weight once you are in the maintenance phases (Phases 3 and 4) is a "correction day" or, more commonly a "steak day." The instructions I'd been given told me to weigh myself every morning before doing anything, and if my weight ever went even slightly more than two pounds over my last injection weight (LIW), to do a "steak day" immediately.

According to my nutritionist, on a "steak day," or "correction day," I was to go the entire day drinking only water (I was allowed some coffee too), and then finish the day with a huge steak and a raw tomato.

Now, I completely understand that this may not seem like (or be) a healthy practice, and if you're of that opinion, I agree with you. In your maintenance phases, and for the rest of your life, your goal needs to be getting the right nutrition and activity on a daily basis so that you never need to do a "steak day" just to maintain your goal weight. I think the highly beneficial part of doing steak days is that it causes you to closely monitor weight fluctuations and take action when those fluctuations occur! You may choose to use a "steak day" (if recommended by your nutritionist) to deal with those fluctuations, or you may choose to just do a day of low-calorie, nutritious eating. Regardless, my opinion is that the strength of a "correction day" lies in your heightened level of awareness and compulsion to act, and not in any particular food combination.

I personally was fairly disciplined in Phase 3, but I did have days when my body was adjusting to the new caloric intake that my weight would pop up above the threshold. When this happened, I followed the instructions and immediately did a steak day. These were extremely helpful to me!

I quickly discovered that if I went above that two-pound threshold, even one steak day would bring me far below my LIW, and I'd be just fine.

At first, it was scary when I went two pounds over my LIW because I was worried that I was on a track to "gain it all back." Then, after a few times doing correction days, I realized that I felt more empowered than I had ever felt!

In previous weight loss programs, I would either worry that a small increase in weight was going to lead to a big increase in weight, or I wouldn't worry *enough* about my small increase in weight, thinking I was doing fine. With HCG, I was at the wheel, in the driver's seat, finally! I realized that it *was* important to pay attention to small increases in weight, but that I was completely in control and able to handle those increases by doing a correction day. I found that it felt very powerful to know that I would wake up daily and, if I saw that I was increasing, know how to fix it myself. Once I got into the cycle of eating good foods in Phase 3, I realized I wouldn't need to do this often, but when I did, I could have confidence knowing I'd be back at a healthy weight the next day.

Here's a word of caution on steak days. Make sure to wake up really early if you think you have a steak day coming. If you think you've eaten something wrong and you're going to be up a couple of pounds tomorrow, *plan to wake up early*, no matter what. *Force it.* That's because, at the end of a steak day, you're going to feel a bit funny and, if you're like me, you're going to be craving breads and starches. You'll want to eat a potato and a basket of bread with that steak. My advice is to get the steak day over with and get to sleep before you binge! The earlier you rise, the more likely it will be that you can make this happen.

I found that I came to enjoy steak days and not stress out about them at all when I needed to do them. When you've gotten through a tough day at work and you get to look forward to a nice, big steak, life isn't so bad!

Again, I'm excited because I'm now armed with the tools I need to maintain my weight. I feel like I'm powerful. I know that my weight will *not* go up, because I won't let it. If it starts to rise, I know exactly how to get it back down. I know how much I can "cheat," because I've experimented. I know what I should eat daily, I know what will happen if I eat other things, and I know how to correct things if they get out of hand. It's an amazing feeling. Though I'm not likely to cheat – because I don't want to test the system and I don't want to *have* to do a correction day – I'm much more comfortable taking off on a vacation or changing up my schedule for a day now, because I'm not afraid I'll lose control or my newfound belt size.

ESTABLISHING A "SET POINT"

IN YOUR READING ABOUT HCG, you may find talk of your body having a "set point." This is described as a naturally-occurring weight your body "gets used to," making it difficult for your body to deviate from that weight. For example, if your body is at 200 pounds, it can be very difficult to get it to go below (but also above) that weight. It's like we're all living at a plateau at whatever weight we're at. This can help us or hurt us. When we get overweight and want to lose weight, this "set point" makes it feel like it's impossible to do so. However, when we reach a new weight that we're happy with and we're able to create a new "set point" at that weight, it can help us!

Medical research shows that this "set point" phenomenon exists, and in my experience, that's absolutely true.[70] Once I had spent over a month at my new body weight in Phase 3, it felt like it was impossible to break it. I had been more and more consistently weighing in at 193.5, my LIW, and the graphs I was keeping on my iPhone looked better and better – more and more within this very tight channel between 193.1 and 193.7. I'd almost never go out of that range, no matter what went into my mouth.

I did get a little cocky because of this. One day I went to the movies and had popcorn and tater tots. (I know – tater tots at a theater? Yep. Come to Scottsdale, Arizona, and go to iPic – it's awesome.) I felt like it was a real treat and I loved every bite, because I'd done so well over the last week. I expected my weight to blow up – nope. It actually went *down* very slightly. I noticed the dots on my trend line were right near each other – I was leveling out. I had my new set point after about a month. For a long time, no matter what I would eat, my body would maintain that set point at 193. It became tough to make my weight budge up or down from there (other than hydration types of factors).

This is exciting! Once you get to your new set point, you'll find that you're actually able to live a much more normal life at your new weight. You'll still always need to keep a lookout for anything that's two pounds over that LIW and plan to do a steak day no matter what when that happens, but otherwise, you may find that you're able to eat a lot of things you didn't think you could eat, without going outside of that range. It's liberating! Now, when your friend has some candy, you can have some, too. You have the tools to stay at your new weight.

I will say this about my weight: The one thing I found I need to be careful with, because it will cause big fluctuations, is cheese. Even a little cheese causes me to retain water and food in my system and causes weight gain. A lot of cheese (say, if I were to order a Chicago-style pizza one time) might cause me to gain four to five pounds in a day, thereby forcing a steak day upon me. Now that I know this about myself, I really stay on the lookout for cheeses and I avoid them at all costs. It's just not worth it to me. Now, even if I'm in on a pizza order on the weekend, I order a thin crust with just veggies, no cheese, and light sauce. This tends to be just fine and not affect my weight. If I get the cheese on there, it may force a steak day tomorrow, and doing that again and again is just not healthy.

FINDING VARIETY IN PHASE 4

PHASE 4 IS SLIGHTLY different from Phase 3, in that you'll continue to eat healthy foods (and eat a lot of them) but you'll begin to add various foods in that weren't on the plan during Phase 3, so you can see how your body responds to them.

This is the time to expand, explore, and build variety into your diet!

This can be one of the most rewarding parts of the HCG diet plan, because it's when you get to turn into a "normal person" again, while operating at your new, lower weight!

One of the basic human needs, though it might surprise you, is variety. You need variety. You can't eat the same stuff every day without starting to become interested in other foods. If you eat the same thing every day, you'll want other things.

So, thinking about systems, as we discussed above, apply that to foods. You need to find foods that taste good to you, that fit into your system. Once you've done that, you need to expand and find a variety of foods to choose from that all taste good and that all fit into your system.

If there's any one of your foods that you hate and won't eat on a daily basis, chuck it. You won't eat it for life. It's a "diet" food for you, and that's no good.

Phase 4 is the time to experiment and find the *widest variety* of nutritious foods that you *actually* can see yourself eating for life. While in Phase 2, you had to keep it strict to lose the weight, and that was fine. Once Phases 3 and 4 come around, it's time to branch out! Throw in one or two foods you haven't tried and find all sorts of different spices, oils, and combinations you can make.

The more foods you find now that fit into your system, the less likely you'll be to consider this a "diet" and "go off" of it someday.
Creating this variety will highly increase the likelihood that this plan will fit into the rest of your life.

Here are some examples of ways that I expanded as I began to eat correctly and cook for myself.

I started off in Phase 2 just with green apples as fruit, plain chicken for protein, and asparagus for my vegetable. After I got into Phase 3, I started to expand my diet by adding in lean ground turkey for my protein and bell peppers and onions. I added tomatoes and mushrooms and kept going from there. My favorite and most convenient meal, by far, is lettuce wraps, which I'll tell you more about in the "Weight Loss Saviors" section.

When I started out on my plan, I tried to use my Vitamix to blend various juices, thinking I'd be really healthy doing that. For me, it's just not sustainable. I didn't like the juices enough to keep drinking them, so I found other ways to eat the veggies, like including them in sauces for my mini-pizzas or in omelets and lettuce wraps. That's when I really started to expand my options.

I found that I craved pizza but (in the spirit of "knowing myself") I dug deeper to figure out that what I craved was mostly the taste of the tomato sauce, not necessarily the cheese or the bread. I found a low-sugar tomato sauce and baked whole wheat tortillas in the oven to make them like thin crusts (but very low-calorie). Then I'd put a *ton* of vegetables, like onions, peppers, tomatoes, mushrooms, and olives, on the top, and just a tiny bit of cheese (only if my weight was in the right range and I knew I could sustain a little weight retention overnight). These little pizzas are now one of my favorite things to make. They're very nutritious, they cure my pizza craving, they're very low in calories, and they deliver a lot of veggie servings in one sitting.

I will caution you HCG users to remember we're talking about Phase 4 at this point. As I said earlier, do not try these veggie pizzas in Phase 2! I did, and it was a big mistake. The veggie pizzas, with their cheese, sauce, and starchy tortilla crusts, didn't cause me to gain weight, but if I snuck them in, they absolutely caused me to plateau. I don't recommend these as a weight loss food, but I do recommend them for Phase 3 and Phase 4. I especially recommend having some of these on standby if you're a guy like me (or Derrick) who craves pizza sometimes.

I also started to drink other beverages, like adding some naturally flavored sparkling waters instead of sodas. I found that I had entirely kicked my energy drink habit at this point. I had also gotten rid of my taste for sweetener and cream in coffee and was now perfectly satisfied with black coffee. To give myself an occasional "treat," I started drinking La Croix sparkling waters, which are naturally flavored and have very few calories. I wouldn't use these as my major source of water, but I found that they're a nice treat if you've been drinking healthy amounts of water all day.

Though you may think that drinking diet sodas is okay because they contain very few calories, research indicates that you should avoid this option. An article published in the *Health Education Journal* showed that diet sodas are actually correlated to higher Body Mass Index (BMI), and that they have been shown to promote weight gain.[71] If your nutritionist suggests that you use these in some way, I can't advise against it, but I would suggest that if you decide together that it isn't the best option, that you consider adding sparkling water to the mix while trying to kick the soda habit.

In all of my testing, I found a few meals that I could always prepare and that I'm sure I'll enjoy for life, while maintaining variety and staying happy. The list below is just a starting point for you. I encourage you to explore the thousands of options available online, including the many HCG cookbooks available on Amazon, and to experiment until you find a balance of variety and convenience that suits your tastes and lifestyle.

- Lettuce wraps

- Omelets

- Spaghetti (using a slicer that turns squash into noodles)

- Fajitas without the shell

- Grilled Chicken Strips with Salsa or Mustard

This is enough to get me through the week. I, of course, still have pieces of fish, steak, and chicken. The ideas above just allow me to branch out from those without taking up a lot of time. More importantly, for each of the items above, I can cook for days in advance and keep them stored. This makes them great for taking to work in a storage container, even if I don't have a lot of time to cook on a given day.

VACATION SETBACKS

I SHOULDN'T COMPLETE MY story of the journey without telling you about the cruise I went on. In Phase 4, after leveling out at my LIW weight for over two months, I took a cruise. Whoops.

I'll say this: Cruises are one of the *best* places in the world to eat great nutritious foods. You're surrounded by the bad but also the good. For breakfast, there are hard-boiled eggs already prepared and ready to eat! There's fruit spread out everywhere. There's cottage cheese. There's fresh coffee at all times. You can even order huge bottles of water from any server you see! It can be a great place to relax and indulge in great healthy foods without veering from the plan if you choose.

However...

It's *very difficult* for Derrick to eat any of that stuff when he's also totally surrounded by cakes, pies, pizzas, cheese, noodles, sugary Jimmy Buffett "boat drinks," and 24-hour free room service. Yes, all of this was included in the price of the cruise package we purchased!

I found myself struggling with temptation throughout the cruise. If you get on a cruise ship and only eat the good stuff, you have *will of iron* that I just do not possess. As much as I thought that, because I had reached Phase 4 and had such success so far, I could just behave, I really struggled. I ended up doing my fair share of bad eating on that boat.

Would I go on another cruise? Probably not – unless I was *very* conditioned to the weight I wanted to be at.

The good news is, I learned something about myself. I know now that as much as I think I'm immune to temptation from having been at my LIW for this long, I'm not. I still need to make sure that I keep my habits adjusted! For the rest of my life, it will probably need to be early to bed, early to rise, and stay on the plan through the day as much as I can. I think that's fine and I'm totally accustomed to it. I just need to be very careful of extended periods of time with tons of food all around me for free. Even a place that wasn't all-inclusive would have helped. I was fine at the Hotel del Coronado, but the all-you-can-eat environment with temptations and sweet boat drinks everywhere can really be an enabler, and I found that I need to be more careful about the temptations I expose myself to.

I also discovered on the cruise that even though my body reached a new "set point," it was *not* invincible. After one day of eating the cruise food, I was fine (I actually brought a scale). After two, I was not fine. After three, I was way up in weight. I needed to do a steak day on the cruise and, after that, I really struggled to maintain the right foods the rest of the seven-day vacation. I ended up having to work extra hard when we returned from the cruise to get back to my LIW and stay there consistently for a while.

It was quite the struggle, and going through it with my nutritionist for a few weeks was frustrating. In the end, about a month after the cruise, I was back to consistently cooking and eating the right things, visiting the nutritionist, and staying within two pounds of my LIW. It was not worth it.

My recommendation to you, if you choose to do this kind of a plan, is that in the early stages, just don't tempt yourself. Do your best to maintain your health and your schedule, add in exercise, and focus on stabilization. Don't think you're invincible. Just because you look good in a bathing suit now doesn't mean you're ready to go to an all-you-can-eat buffet!

KNOWING THYSELF: BAD SCENARIOS

AS YOU'VE NOW LEARNED, cruises are a bad place for me. This is worth further discussion.

The cruise, for me, was a setback, but also a good learning opportunity. I learned about myself. Every time you learn about yourself, you get stronger. I learned cruises enable me and are a bad place. You learn what your bad places are. You recover. You forgive yourself. You move forward.

I also know that car trips are a bad place for me.

To succeed, you need to find your bad places and avoid them like the plague.

There are certain scenarios that will bring you down. I personally have found that I can't seem to travel yet without screwing up. Even though I hope to travel more someday, I recognize my current limitations, and this is one of them. When I hit the road, Derrick comes out and starts making excuses about what he should be able to eat "just for this one day."

Part of this process is changing yourself so you're ready for anything. However, another part of the process, as we've discussed, is knowing yourself so well that you understand what situations you can do well in and what situations will cause you to fail.

Someone building a new house wants to build it so it's ready to weather ice storms. But that doesn't mean that as soon as the wooden frame is up, they just yell out to the sky, "Bring on the hail!" It takes many months of framing and roofing before that house is ready for that kind of storm. Heck, even when that storm comes at a prepared house, some repairs might still be needed afterward.

Don't put yourself in a hailstorm before you're ready. Realize your limitations and be very intentional about not putting yourself in a place to take a direct hit. Even the best boxers don't want to get punched right in the face! Keep your guard up, even when you know you're strong. For me, that meant not going to bars and restaurants after work, not taking long car trips when possible, and *no cruises with free food*!

Sure, I should be able to do these things but, honestly, I can't. Eventually, I'll mess up. Someone will *buy* me that shot that I didn't want to drink, and a great friend will convince me I should stay for that one "last beer." The influences around you will find a way to draw you back into your bad habits. Friends may hurt your progress, even though they don't mean to. Even people who love you can wreck your plans without meaning any harm. Just like the drowning victim isn't an evil person, intent on drowning the lifeguard, he can still easily do so while reaching out for anything that floats!

Learn what your temptations are. Learn when you're likely to fail. Learn about your bad spots, and use that knowledge to your advantage! Do everything you can to avoid the scenarios that make you do the bad things, then get yourself away from them.

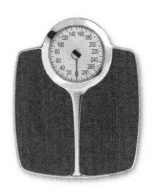

PART 5:
THE BEST ADVICE
I CAN GIVE YOU

WHAT FOLLOWS IS A list of the best advice I can give you so that you are successful in your transformation. Take notes about the ideas that you feel you can apply to your life!

BEST ADVICE I CAN GIVE YOU: USING YOUR STRONG TIMES

PART OF KNOWING THYSELF is knowing when your energy levels are greatest. Pay great attention to this time of day – whenever it may be – and make sure that, during that time of day, you are ready to accomplish what you want to accomplish. Whether that is important projects at work, cooking, working out – whatever is most important to you, you should plan to do it when you have your highest natural levels of focus and energy.

I find that my highest levels of focus and energy occur about one to two hours after waking up and only carry through until about 11:00 A.M. I know that sounds absurd.

You're thinking, *Really Eric? You only have high energy and focus from 7:00 to 11:00 A.M.?*

I answer, yes. And, because I know myself well, I can get enough done between those hours that I don't need to really do much that requires absolute focus and energy for the rest of the day.

When I really take an honest assessment of each day's achievements, I find that the real work got done in a small subsection of the day – usually lasting only an hour at most. I make big progress in little time, and the rest of the day is often spent firefighting.

Perhaps there are experts on personal energy who can offer me ways to widen this time and be productive longer, but honestly, I get a *lot* done in that sprint time. I pound through more work in those four hours than most people do in a day or two. I know myself well, I plan to use that energy wisely, I make sure I'm not distracted during that time, and, because of it (not being cocky here – just telling you what actually happened), I was able to maintain my work as an executive while getting an MBA, losing 30 pounds, spending Friday nights playing guitar at a restaurant, and writing this book. I got a lot done this year, and most days I did that in tiny windows of focus – tiny "sprints" – which I took advantage of when I felt a burst of energy coming on. I didn't do all of this by grinding for 24 hours straight. I did my fair share of burning the midnight oil and the early morning oil, but when I felt tired, I rested, and when I felt energized, I took advantage of the opportunity. I challenge anyone who thinks they're really "on point" all day to take an honest assessment and decide whether that's true or whether their big achievements happened in small sprints.

Whatever truth you find, know thyself and then use that knowledge!

I wrote this whole chapter in eight minutes. I didn't plan this time of the day – I just made sure I was at my desk, doing productive things, during this time of strength. By positioning myself this way to face the day, this chapter just kind of got written – I just turned to the computer and banged it out – quickly! I think it would be a mistake to plan the day to a "T" and try to schedule writing for a time when I know I will be tired. Derrick will find something else to do during that time.

Instead of doing that, I have my list of important priorities to tackle, and I keep that list with me. I block my strong time on my calendar so I can focus during that time on what matters most. During that sprint, I'll easily write a chapter a day, without even planning specifically for that activity. A *huge* mistake would be to schedule a long, low-impact, boring update meeting during that time. That would rob me of my time of strength. Sure, I'd be alert and highly participative at that meeting, but I'd burn my chances of really getting things done that day, because I'd be out of my productive zone later in the day when the work needed to get done. For that reason, I try to get meetings off of my calendar during my times of strength.

There will be certain "strong times" that come unexpectedly. This may happen to you at 8:00 P.M. on a Friday, when you thought you would be exhausted! When those moments of productivity hit you, I strongly advise that you use them!

When you feel inspired to go – GO!

Sometimes, at random, I'll hit a strong time and, all of a sudden, I'll be racing around my condo doing laundry, cooking, and writing papers for school. When this happens, I use that energy! Likewise, there are a lot of times when I have a list of things to do and I am not feeling strong. When that happens, as long as the results won't be catastrophic, I sit still. When you're tired and compelled to sit still, do that. But, in return for that, when you're feeling high-energy and compelled to get a few things done – let that take you! Get them done! Fly around knocking things out! Right now, I'm in a strong time – it's now 7:58 A.M. In eight minutes, I've written this entire chapter. I'm off to be strong doing something else!

BEST ADVICE I CAN GIVE YOU: IF YOU HAVE THE TIME, USE IT FOR COOKING

I'VE SPENT A LOT of time in my life exercising – sometimes up to two and a half hours a day, trying to lose weight. I've found that if I have only a limited amount of time in the morning to get anything done, it's much, much more productive for me to use that time to cook healthy food for the day than it is for me to cram in a workout. I could go to the gym, sweat it out, not lose a pound, then go around scrounging for food all day and maybe eat some wrong things ... or I could spend that same amount of time cooking *amazing* food –even if it requires an early morning trip to the grocery store – and eating all the right things later that day.

People say, "I don't have time to cook." I used to say it, too, yet I'd use my free time to work out. Looking back, it puzzles me: My goal was to lose weight, yet I'd spend all of my time focused on workouts and tell my nutritionist, "I don't have time to cook." My thought now is, "I don't have time to exercise, because I have to cook!"

Get this, in a study published in the *Journal of Consumer Affairs,* people who read food labels who did not exercise displayed a greater likelihood of weight loss than those who exercised but did not read food labels![72] Food makes a huge difference! If you're spending all of your time on the treadmill and none in the kitchen or at the grocery store, you may want to rethink your priorities.

Doesn't it seem like it's hard to get good food without heading to the grocery store? It's just hard to find. If you're going to a restaurant or a deli or, honestly, anywhere that's not a grocery store, you're taking a risk that you don't know what's in the food or how it is prepared.

In my experience, no matter what I'm looking for, even if I find it, it always seems to have some bad stuff in it.

When I manage to find yogurt at a cafe, it always seems to be some high-fat yogurt parfait with some sort of sugar-added fruit goo in it.

Find somewhere to grab some eggs? Guess what – they come with cheese and were cooked in a ton of oil.

Want some veggies? They're probably covered in cheese and sauce.

Want soup? They put whole cream in that one for consistency. It's very hard to make good decisions when there's so much bad content in the food that's prepared in restaurants.

Want a sandwich? That much bread – no way. And the lunch meat is full of preservatives.

Here's the thing, if you don't want to look like a "normal" person then you shouldn't eat what everyone thinks is normal. Normal, these days, is obese. If you eat what they eat, you're going to look like them. If you want to look different, you can't eat what's normal. You have to learn to prepare your foods and eat healthy foods. People will think that's weird, and the norm is that you should be able to eat what people around you seem to be eating, but you can't. Most people don't like the feeling that they're doing something different from everyone else, because they feel like it's not normal. Let the "normal" continue on with their lives the way they feel comfortable. You're going to do things that make you uncomfortable, because you know that's the only way you can create change.

BEST ADVICE I CAN GIVE YOU: CHECK YOUR WEIGHT IN THE MORNING

THIS ALMOST GOES WITHOUT saying, but I need to say it anyway. You should weigh yourself every single morning, as soon as you get up, right after "evacuating" anything in your system. This is the most consistent way to monitor your weight, and you can trust it. Don't weigh yourself through the day, because you'll be very inconsistent even within an hour of waking up, depending on what you've had to eat and drink. Instead, look forward to this one morning weigh-in as the time when you gauge your progress.

I have heard the arguments that weighing-in every morning may be disheartening because it's possible that you may not see significant progress, and might even see a small gain day-over-day. I personally would rather know the truth at all times. If I gain a little weight, I would rather know it right away and take action, than wait another day without making an adjustment or at least being very aware of my water and food intake for the day. I'm not an ostrich, burying my head in the sand pretending the weight gain doesn't exist. If there's a problem, I want to know about it, face it, and take action to fix it. If there's not a problem, I want to celebrate it and let my momentum build. I also personally observed that my weight gains and losses were *extremely* consistent with my eating and activity. There are very few (if any) days I can remember, where I executed perfectly on my exercise, hydration, nutrition, and sleep, and ended up seeing a weight gain. On days when I did see a gain, I knew why. On days when I saw a loss, I knew why. Your results may be different, but for me, daily weigh-ins were reflective of my activity, and were helpful.

I now look forward to this morning weigh-in very much. It's "ceremonial." I pop out of bed, anxious to see my progress. People told me this eagerness to get up and weigh in would end after Phase 2, but for me, it didn't. To this day, months after ending my weight loss phase and being in a perpetual state of maintenance, I'm still excited about my weight. I'm still excited to jump into clothes I wouldn't have been able to before, and I'm excited to write in my journal about how my health and wellness are progressing.

I encourage you to weigh yourself in the morning so that you're tracking your progress, so that you know when you might need a steak day, and so that you develop this ceremony. Why? Because the ceremony is fun, and it will keep you on track.

Before you achieve your goal, you'll see your progress here. Sometimes you'll cheat, and you'll see the effect of your cheating; this ceremony will help you to put the bad actions behind you. You'll weigh in, you'll be up a pound or two (or four), you'll forgive yourself, and you'll move on to another healthy day. The next day, you'll be back on track. On great days, you'll literally cheer, and on even days you'll smile happily. It's a good schedule to get on, and I highly recommend it. Your new morning ceremony is to pop up and weigh in.

BEST ADVICE I CAN GIVE YOU: STAY HYDRATED

WE HAVE ALL HEARD about the importance of staying hydrated. It keeps you healthy, it keeps you from overeating, and it's something almost nobody does well. Your nutritionist will most likely suggest that you drink more water than you're used to. I completely agree. You might as well just refer to this stuff as "skinny juice." Here are some ideas that stemmed from my attempts to stay hydrated.

I work at a place where there are a lot of meetings. I hate to admit it, but these meetings are tough to pay attention in, and they last forever. I have found, though, that these meetings are a chance to become very well hydrated. As I sit and sometimes participate in the meetings, I bring bottles of water with me and challenge myself to get the entire bottle down by the end of the meeting.

This does two things for me. First, it keeps me hydrated. Second, it sometimes gets me out of the meeting for a few minutes when I need to get rid of the excess hydration in the men's room.

Either way, I've now developed a phrase I swear by:

"Every boring meeting is another chance to keep yourself hydrated."

It's now the norm to grab a bottle of water on the way out the door to the meeting and make sure that bottle is finished by the end!

I encourage you to find activities where you can get a bottle of water in. Could it be your morning drive to work? Your evening drive home? Waiting for your son or daughter at the bus stop or after school? Wherever it may be, I encourage you to develop these little "hydration rituals" and let them be reminders to you about when to bring along a bottle of water and when to stay hydrated.

If you're bored by the flavor of water, ask your nutritionist about adding a little bit of fresh lemon juice. During this program, I bought a little lemon juicer that I used to extract fresh juice from lemons to add to water. I ended up not using it much. It was time consuming and the lazy Derrick in me would rather do without the taste than take the time to buy and squeeze lemons.

While we're talking water, I have two other points to make that are important.

One, you should always have a ton of water with you, and have both cold and room-temperature water. I personally stock my car with two cases of San Pellegrino at all times. I also have a case at home and a case in the office, but I also keep an *extra* two cases in the car, so that at *any time* I have it available to me. As long as my car is outside, whether I'm at a hotel, restaurant, meeting, anywhere, I can grab water. I also make sure I'm stocked with room-temperature still water – just regular spring water from the bottle, because it's easier to chug one of those than a sparkling water if I'm feeling dehydrated. I keep both warm and cold bottles of sparkling and still water around me, in case I'm in the mood for one or the other.

Second, if you're the kind of person who makes a fuss about our use of too many bottles of water, that's fine. Buy a ton of your big, environmentally-friendly containers and use them! Again, *get a ton of them.* Put them everywhere and get in the habit of refilling them all the time.

Don't land in the middle, where you don't buy enough and don't drink enough. The mission here is to stay hydrated!

I'm not judging you, no matter which side of the water bottle argument you're on. I am judging you if you don't find ways to get enough water in you.

Whatever your preference is on water bottles, get a ton of them and drink water all the time.

On a final note, I'll admit that I used to be worried about drinking too much water because I thought it would cause me to weigh-in higher on the scale! This was, of course, short-term thinking and counterproductive. I now have found that when I drink more water in a day, I have a much greater chance of weighing less the next morning. By not drinking enough water, I often find that I retain more weight and weigh in higher! If you find that you're not weighing in where you should, yet you're eating right, focus on how much water you had the previous day. Try to get more of it before you assume you just ate the wrong foods.

BEST ADVICE I CAN GIVE YOU: THINK OF OPTIONS BEFORE OPPOSITION

I FIND THAT THE most successful people I know are always thinking of ways to make things happen. I also find that the biggest failures I know are people who are always telling you why things can't happen. In the case of your nutrition and, honestly, any area of your life, it's critical that you figure out ways to make things happen. As you listen to the advice I'm giving you, you may hear a voice in your head saying, *Yes, that will work for me!* You may also hear voices in your head saying, *No, that would never work for me – he doesn't get it.* If you're the latter, you're thinking the wrong way.

You need to be thinking about *how* to make things work, not about why things won't work.

So fine, your car can't hold two cases of water because you drive a motorcycle to work. It's time to sign up for grocery delivery.

You may be thinking, *I can't afford all this bottled water.* Guess what? One-gallon jugs of water are 69 cents. Drink those. I sometimes just buy one of those and carry it around with me all day until it's gone, instead of drinking the bottles. It's cheaper and uses less plastic; plus, they're easily refillable.

You may be thinking, *I live deep in the woods, and there are no nutritionists out here.* Fine Thoreau, go online where you got this book and sign up for online help from one of the chat services that offers professional legal and behavioral services without leaving your computer.

Find options – get creative.

If you're the kind of person who's always thinking and talking about why things won't ever work, you need to change that. If you don't get away from that way of thinking, you're likely to fail at everything you try, including this transformation. Also, if you don't get away from that way of thinking, people will probably always think you're miserable to be around. It's true.

During my transformation, I spoke with someone who was also interested in losing some weight. He wanted advice on a protein to eat that was portable that didn't require cooking.

"Cottage cheese," I said.

"I can't," he said, "I can't have dairy."

I went on to mention other options, each of which he said was difficult or impossible for him to do. This conversation showed me that his mind wasn't in the place it needed to be for him to be successful. He was thinking of every way to say no and no ways to say yes.

Someone in the right mindset would have said, "You know, that's not a bad idea. I have trouble with cottage cheese, but do you know of other proteins like that – is there a non-dairy equivalent to cottage cheese?" My friend wasn't in the right state of mind yet to accept advice. Also, by looking for options outside of cooking, he was showing that he wasn't ready to invest the time to make a change. Inside, he was still not open to the idea of changing his life, and therefore he wasn't open to working with me to figure out options.

He wanted my validation that this program would not work for him, and I would not give him that validation. All I would do was continue to give him options, until he realized that *his thinking* was the problem.

No matter what you want to do, if you care enough, you can find a way.

Regardless of the problem at hand, there is always a solution if there is a passionate thinker, ready to propose options. Think of options. Until you become a person who can convince himself or herself how to do things, you will remain a person who convinces himself or herself that things cannot be done, and you will never succeed.

To my friend's credit, not being ready isn't necessarily a bad thing. There will be a time in his life where this becomes important enough to him to make the big changes that need to be made. The problem is not that he is unable to change, but instead that he is attempting to start something before he is ready to commit. Personal transformation is not something to be casually hoped for – it must be truly strived for!

A great mentor of mine often quotes the Buddhist Proverb, "when the student is ready, the teacher will appear." When you are ready to think of options, as opposed to opposition, the options will come to you in many ways.

BEST ADVICE I CAN GIVE YOU: CREATE SUSTAINABLE SYSTEMS

I MENTIONED THIS BEFORE when speaking about habits and identity, and now I'm going to go deeper into it.

To create lasting change, make sure anything you do is sustainable, and repeatable.

If it's not sustainable and repeatable, it's not worth doing. I always get irritated when someone tells me about their super healthy meal or super healthy day. An unhealthy person I know once told me, "I spent all day yesterday cooking these healthy foods, and now today I have all of my healthy meals all ready to go." I laughed to myself, because I knew this was the kind of person that would do this once and would never do it again. *That's great*, I thought, *but what about tomorrow, or the next day, or the day after that? What are you going to do this week and next week?*

If you can't repeat your behavior enough to turn it into a habit that can be practiced daily, it will have

virtually no impact on your life. You need to create repeatable, sustainable systems.

Success in Phase 3 and Phase 4 has everything to do with this concept. As I mentioned previously, it took some time for me to get used to bringing the right foods in to work with me. At first I was carrying way too much, and in the end, I found a way to create a sustainable, repeatable system that allowed me to do this daily without it being a nuisance. Did I quit? Did I give up? Nope. Many people, when faced with adversity, would say, "Nobody can do this in real life, it's too hard." Instead, I created a *system* that could easily work for the rest of my life.

Preparing for a major life (and schedule) change ahead of time might just help you stay on track when the change comes. For example, as I would try out changes to my habits, I used the following test. As I would try preparing a new meal, or add a new activity to my calendar, even though I don't have kids, I would think, *if I had to do this and also pack kids' lunches in the morning, could I do it?* If the answer was no, I needed to improve the system. If the answer was yes, I was doing well. Some of you who do have kids and who do pack lunches for them have no choice but to go by this advice.

Don't wear yourself out in one day, thinking that you could never sustain that behavior. Instead, always think in terms of systems – sustainable, repeatable actions, that can turn into habits, that can become "second nature," that don't take over your life and make you think of this as temporary, and you'll have a much greater chance of succeeding in the long term.

BEST ADVICE I CAN GIVE YOU: THE POWER OF RHYTHM AND CLEARING WEEKENDS

ALONG THE LINES OF sustainable systems, I also think it's important that you create extra time, or "padding," during which you can make sure your systems are in order. This often means clearing time, specifically on nights and weekends, to take care of things that aren't currently planned for.

Here's something I know about myself. I know that if I don't buy groceries and do laundry on weekends, I'll have almost no time to do those things on weekdays and I'll end up foregoing those activities and stressing out about them all week. I know, because of this, that it's critical for me to make time on weekends to get these things done. Therefore, I'm very, very careful about making commitments on weekends.

When people ask, "Can we hang out Saturday?" I really work hard to figure out what we're going to do and when before I commit. Honestly, even though you can call me anti-social, I don't like to even commit to *anything* on weekends anymore.

If I find out at the last minute that I have extra time after doing what I need to, like shopping and laundry, to go out and have some fun then I may make last-minute plans. But there's something about having a full weekend totally free, as Friday night approaches, that lets you truly relax and get your life into the state of productivity that it needs to be in if you want to lose this kind of weight quickly.

As I mentioned, I was working toward my MBA while I did the HCG plan and wrote this book. I needed to spend at least five to six hours per weekend-day writing papers and another three to four hours working on the book. Having plans on a Saturday or Sunday can really stress you out when you have all of that going on anyway. I can only imagine how it will be for those of you with kids to go through this.

I can't personally tell you how to create the space in your life and freedom from distractions that this program requires, but I can tell you that it's important to your success not to overcommit to social and even family events. There will be events that you just can't work around, and if that's the case, as I wrote previously, you'll need to find ways to make this work. Having said this, I challenge you to really examine your week's schedule and decide what needs to stay and what can probably go. If you're honest with yourself, you may find that some things you're doing are setting you up for small failures, and could be avoided with planning and commitment.

My best advice to you is to create a "rhythm" in life. *Try to make life boring!* Get rid of your commitments and events that are coming up, at least until you're well into Phase 4. Turn down any requests for your time that doesn't mean a lot to you. Block off all of your extra weekend time – *all* of your weekend time – for free time with your kids, your work commitments (if you work weekends), and your personal organization. Use this time to get laundry done, to keep your home clean, to keep yourself organized and prepared for the coming week, and to spend any extra time either relaxing or devoted to others in your life. Don't book yourself up so that you have no time for these types of restoring behaviors, because you *need* to take part in them to be successful through your work week, if you have one.

Along with this, hopefully by this point I've convinced you that if you tend to eat more at night, you should be waking up early and going to bed early. If you've chosen to do this, I think you should continue to do this on the weekends, maintaining that rhythm of "early to rise, early to bed," every day. This will make Mondays a lot easier and will allow you to do better with your eating habits through the weekend. Don't convince yourself that you're "giving yourself a break" on Saturdays and Sundays. You can be just as relaxed and rested by getting up early and going to bed early as you would if you woke up late and stayed up late. Honestly, I'll argue that you'll feel more rested with the early riser method.

Use weekend days – or any days you get away from work – to maintain your habit of rising early. Don't let exhaustion on Friday trick you into thinking Saturday you'll be tired. You won't be. Use Saturday and Sunday for you – not to relax, but to move the ball forward!

I'll go further with this line of thinking and say this: While many people think they don't have enough free time, I see enough of it squandered with weekend activities that I've started to think of my weekends as free weekdays.

In other words, there are two weekdays that belong to me: Saturday and Sunday. If I wasted Saturdays and Sundays, like most people do, I would not have been able to complete this transformation, my MBA, or this book.

BEST ADVICE I CAN GIVE YOU: GET TO KNOW THE GROCERY STORE

IF YOU'RE FOLLOWING THE plan your nutritionist has given you and you've begun to cook your own foods, then you're already realizing that you're going to have to spend a lot of time at your local grocery store. Get used to it!

It's important that you find grocery stores that are close to your home and others that are close to where you work. If your default behavior right now, when you get hungry, is to go to a specific restaurant, fast-food joint, or even an at-work cafeteria, you need to change that default behavior to heading out to the grocery store.

Did you come to work without lunch? Time to head to the grocery store.

Is it 8:00 P.M. and you are starving with nothing healthy around? Head to the grocery store.

If you are hungry in any situation and can't find anything to eat, the grocery store is always a better option than a restaurant. Get very, very comfortable with this approach.

During this transformation, I spent many nights headed over to the grocery store instead of doing what I would have done before (as you know, that's ordering pizza). I spent many afternoons popping over to the grocery store from work instead of hitting up the cafeteria or a food truck. My default became the grocery store.

Once this becomes your regular behavior, you'll find that it gets easier and easier. You'll know exactly where your favorite healthy foods are, and you'll be able to pick up what you need very quickly. You'll also start to find that, once you get home, cooking something doesn't take nearly as long as you once would have thought. When you're more practiced with cooking you realize that, within ten minutes, you can brown some meat, add some chopped peppers and spices, and have something delicious and fresh in front of you, as opposed to a burger or a bowl of ice cream.

Use your local grocer to your advantage!

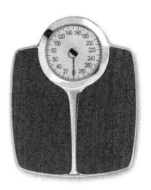

PART 6:
MY WEIGHT LOSS SAVIORS

THERE ARE A FEW things that had such a massive impact on my weight loss journey that I need to call them saviors. I know that's a big word, and I use it with complete sincerity. These things all carried me through the program and, at times, even saved me from making mistakes that could have turned my weight loss in the wrong direction. Here's a list for you.

MY WEIGHT LOSS SAVIORS: COFFEE

I CANNOT SAY ENOUGH good things about coffee. Coffee got me through this program and continues to get me through the day, for many reasons.

First, coffee has almost no calories. You can drink all you want of it and you won't put on weight. Coffee also has flavor, so if you want a treat, it's better than water. To me, coffee is a treat, and it's the one treat we are allowed to have any time. When you wake up in the morning and you feel groggy, coffee is there to get you into the right mindset. When you're trying to adjust your sleep schedule and you force yourself out of bed at 4:00 A.M., coffee makes it possible for you to adjust without being drowsy all morning. I'll add that, when I have caffeine, I'm more alert, I'm pleasant to be around, and I get a ton of things done.

I'll also note that I don't always drink caffeinated coffee. I'd certainly get the jitters if all of the coffee I'm talking about here was full of caffeine! Because I've begun to enjoy coffee's flavor, I also substitute decaf coffee for regular. At the beginning of the program, I drank the decaf stuff a lot, especially at night when I wanted to sleep.

Coffee is also a gourmet item you can indulge in, while you can't participate in others like wine or certain foods. You get to experience a variety of different flavors and become your own version of a coffee sommelier as you learn what you enjoy most. It can be fun, and it's a great way to keep your taste buds active as you don't get to indulge in food as much.

At the very least, coffee is a nice treat to go along with your healthy breakfast. When you're at a restaurant and your friends order dessert, you get to order coffee, and some restaurants have great, great coffee. Treat yourself to it!

Your nutritionist will probably tell you that you should not put sweetener or cream in your coffee. In my program, I was allowed just a tiny bit of milk, but it was so little that I just learned to give that up altogether. I was also allowed stevia-based sweeteners, but I gave those up as well, because by the time I was brave enough to try them, I'd already gotten used to drinking black coffee. To this day, it's what I drink. After time, I didn't miss the cream and Splenda. I started to enjoy trying the different strong blends and appreciated the differences between flavors.

When we were on vacation in Coronado, instead of looking forward to breakfast, I looked forward to a nice morning coffee. When I'd normally order a dessert or a drink, I'd look forward to a new coffee blend. It's a nice treat that's not expensive, and it keeps you on the right path, giving you energy instead of draining you like sugar or alcohol would.

Another benefit to coffee for me was that I used to drink a lot of energy drinks like Red Bull and Monster to get through the workday. I picked up the habit long ago and just never dropped it. Coffee was a way I could keep that caffeine intake going, without the other chemicals, sugars, and sweeteners found in those energy drinks. Even now, long into my Phase 4, I continue to just drink black coffee and have not gone back to energy drinks or to cream and sweeteners. I feel much better through the day, and I love my coffee.

I need to mention that, throughout this process, I used Keurig coffeemakers. I have one at home and one at my office. These coffeemakers make it possible for me to have exactly the kind of coffee I want at any time. If you have the extra cash to grab one or two of these, I highly recommend it. When you get that impulse to eat, you can replace it with a drink of coffee, even if it's decaf, and these Keurig one-cup coffeemakers make that possible.

I also recommend that you add disposable coffee cups to your grocery list. Again, if you're the type of person who wants to save the planet and use a reusable cup, that's fine – make sure you have lots of those and they're clean. If you're not one of those people, then just spend the five dollars on a pack of about 25 disposable cups so that when you want to hit the road with a coffee, one is ready to go.

MY WEIGHT LOSS SAVIORS: OVER-THE-COUNTER SLEEP AIDS

I WILL ADMIT THAT when I first began to get used to the new sleep schedule, I allowed myself to be aided by over-the-counter sleep medicine. If there was a day when I had woken up at 4:00 A.M. yet still wasn't tired enough by about 8:00 P.M. to go to sleep, then I'd take one of these sleep aids to make sure I was in bed and asleep in time to do it again the next day. Though I did this, I did not do it regularly, and I wouldn't advise that you do this without talking to your doctor about the approach. I did discuss this approach with my nutritionist, and she said that as long as I did it sparingly, it might make sense for me in the short-term (considering my late-night binging habit).

I include this information for two reasons. First, because I want to be very honest with you about how I made this change happen in my life, and this was a part of it. Second, because I think that, if your doctor agrees with it, getting some help with going to bed at a decent hour may help you out if you are at all like I was. See, my biggest weight gain problem, by far, was late-night eating. Before I started on this prescriptive plan, I wouldn't get enough nutrition through the day, so I'd binge at about 8:00 or 9:00 P.M. on whatever I could get my hands on, and I loved the feeling of "being full" and falling asleep. Usually, this meant that I would order a pizza from a delivery service at night. Changing my diet didn't make this habit go away immediately, and I was still hungry many nights during Phase 2. So, on those nights, I would anticipate this binging ahead of time, take a dose of the sleep aid, and be out like a light by 9:00 P.M. That way, I wouldn't binge. The next thing I knew, I'd be standing on the scale, one to two pounds lighter than the day before, smiling and proud, ready for another day where my clothes fit better.

After doing this sparingly, I was able to adjust my sleep schedule to one where I arose early and fell asleep early, every day. I'm now living a very healthy lifestyle, I'm no longer in need of the sleep aids, and I'm usually awake from about 4:00 A.M. to about 8:30 P.M. daily.

There are many arguments against the use of these sleep aids, and I can't disagree with any of them! I'm certainly not saying what I did was healthy, or recommending it. I personally concluded that if taking a dose of a sleep aid would allow me to get to bed earlier and wake up earlier, thereby keeping me from eating an extra pizza and giving me a chance to adjust my sleep cycle so that over time I would eat *far* fewer pizzas, it was worth it. For me, the behavioral benefit outweighed the downsides to the approach. There are many natural options out there to help you sleep, including herbal remedies, teas, etc.

I also need to add this: In the end, the sleep aids *were not* the best way for me to form the habit of going to bed early. The best way to do this for me, by far, was to wake up at 4:00 A.M. and not nap at all through the day. This was a much more powerful way to change my habits than to use sleep aids at night. Not to mention, sleep aids sometimes caused residual drowsiness for me, because they'd stay in my system longer than I wanted them to. If you have the discipline to get your behind out of bed at 4:00 A.M. for a few days in a row, without napping at all, I recommend that as the most effective way to adjust your sleep cycle and prefer it over the use of sleep aids. I personally reserved the sleep aids for nights when I just didn't feel tired enough to get to bed early, and felt that a binge might be coming my way if I didn't end up asleep on time.

MY WEIGHT LOSS SAVIORS: FOOD STORAGE CONTAINERS

I'VE FOUND THAT WHEN eating healthy, food storage containers are worth their weight in gold. Buy as many as you can, in many different shapes and sizes. Get tiny ones for dressing, huge ones for full days of omelets and the innards of lettuce wraps. Get medium-sized ones for meats and veggies. Get split ones for your starches. Buy them all!

The more of these containers you have, the more prepared you will be to buy as much food as you need for a full week, keep that food fresh, take that food to work, chop that food up, and keep it until you need it later on.

You need to be able to keep your leftovers and use them later. You need to be able to store yogurt on the way to work. You need to be able to chop up a pepper and keep half of it if you don't use the whole thing. If you only have one or two storage containers, that's hard to do. If you have a hundred storage containers, there is always one on-hand, it's never stuck with the dirty dishes, and you can use it when you need it.

My advice on water bottles and food storage containers is the same. You can't have too many on reserve.

Along with storage containers, get some plastic freezer bags. These are great for separating out your meats. It's likely you'll buy chicken or steak in a pack containing many pieces. When you get home from the store, take some time to separate these out into freezer bags, and then freeze or refrigerate them. This makes things a lot easier later on when it's time to cook.

A neat trick I learned to go along with this storage strategy is that in only about 30 minutes, a steak will thaw out if it's in a freezer bag, and then placed in water. I combine my tools to make this work for me!

Here's how it works. Grab one of your large plastic containers and fill it with water. Put the steak, right in its freezer bag, in the water, and then put the lid on the big container. In 30 minutes, you have a grill-ready steak. This separating-the-meats-into-servings trick, combined with your big storage containers, will give you a way to grill a somewhat quick dinner anytime you're in the mood for a good piece of chicken, fish, or steak!

Containers also make salads really, really easy. I like to bring heads of lettuce with me to work and just chop them up and put them into my containers when I get a break from the action. With salads, some people fear dressing, because it can be very fatty, but I don't. I figure, I'm eating the salad to help control my hunger later, and the most important thing is that I actually eat the salad before Derrick gets hungry and eats something else.

For that reason, I started to use really, really good tasting dressings in Phase 3 and Phase 4. I still do. It's up to you and your doctor, but personally, I'd rather eat a controlled amount of really good dressing that makes me look forward to a salad packed full of veggies, than absolutely dread eating that salad and maybe causing a meal-miss or a binge later. Use tasty dressing in moderation and get that salad into your mouth. Containers help you to do this because you can do one of two things:

1) Grab some tiny containers and use those for your dressings. Pour a pre-determined amount of dressing into these, and when you're eating, dip your fork first into the dressing, then grab a bite of salad.

2) Grab a huge container and put your lettuce in it. Pour a pre-determined amount of dressing into the container with the lettuce, put the top on, and shake like crazy until the dressing is perfectly coating each piece of lettuce.

Using either of the methods above, you have a salad that's going to keep you full for a while and keep Derrick (or whoever your alter-ego is) away from the cravings for that much longer.

Also, reverting back to our talk from the beginning of this book, you need to remember that it's not fatty dressing that ruined our diet plans before – it's our habits that would destroy any diet we try. I found that eating a salad with a good tasting dressing caused me to stay on track, and that my weight gains were attributed to *not* eating during the day and *overeating* at night, more than they were due to eating the wrong foods during the day.

As you now know, this book is about preparing to set yourself up for success, and if some fatty dressing gets you to put a head of lettuce into your mouth before your Derrick takes over and eats 20 sticks of beef jerky, then let's take the dressing.

Your problem isn't that you chose the wrong dressing. Your problem is that you ruin every diet you try.

Along the lines of buying big containers, you're going to find yourself buying a lot of things during this plan that other people just wouldn't buy. You're initially going to think you're crazy when you find yourself buying five heads of lettuce in a week because you want to make lettuce wraps. But here's the thing – you're not crazy. You actually do need five heads of lettuce sometimes, so buy them! It's not expensive, but it is strange. It's going to be bulky. It's going to be a lot to carry. But if you need it for nutrition, buy it. Even though you will find yourself thinking, *Oh this is so weird – nobody buys all of this lettuce*, realize that you need it for nutrition, so buy it.

You may need 15 green peppers for the week. Fine! Buy them! They're like 59 cents! Most people wouldn't buy that many, but honestly, most people are overweight. Most people would buy a box of sugary granola bars. Most people would eat those thinking they're being healthy, while you're eating your veggies and being "strange." Realize that most people are wrong, and that in order to look and feel different than most people you see, you're going to have to act differently than most people, most of the time.

Just remember that most people are wrong, and that you gained weight because you were doing the wrong things. Doing the right things for your health and your weight are going to feel strange to you, because you haven't been doing them. They will also be strange to other people who do not do them. Weird feelings or not, you need to do them. While our friends go to Jamba Juice, taking down a bowl of ice cream blended with some pieces of fruit, we'll be eating veggies. Just remember, they're going to still be chunky, slurping up that Jamba Juice, while you're feeling better than you have in years. Yet, they'll call you weird for bringing in your lunch every day! The world is upside down – never forget that as you progress.

MY WEIGHT LOSS SAVIORS: SAN PELLEGRINO

I'VE LEARNED TO SWEAR by San Pellegrino. I don't remember exactly how or why I began to drink it, but it has been a savior for me. As I've mentioned, I used to drink too many energy drinks and would get a kick out of the flavor, carbonation, and buzz I got from them on a regular basis at work. I found that a great substitute that still delivered the carbonation, but in a beverage that was more healthy, was San Pellegrino spring water. You might want to opt for regular water, but for whatever reason, I craved the carbonation. Regular water just seems boring to me. Give me an ice cold San Pellegrino anytime, and I'll just thank you for it. If your nutritionist allows it, you can even add a bit of fresh lemon juice to the San Pellegrino to give it some flavor!

On a final note, like the Boy Scouts say, "be prepared." If you want to drink seven to eight bottles of water per day, and you do the math, it means you're going to need 49-56 bottles of the stuff per week. If you have less than that, you're not ready for the week.

MY WEIGHT LOSS SAVIORS: GREAT HIGH-END RESTAURANTS

ANOTHER ONE OF MY saviors throughout this weight loss period was high-end restaurants. I was advised by my nutritionist to stay away from restaurants when possible, because they often flavor their food with butter and other things you just don't need in your body. However, I was able to find some restaurants, especially high-end ones, that would prepare foods any way I asked them to. While traveling, this became very helpful!

Even if high-end restaurants may seem very expensive, you may find, as I did, that without ordering any appetizers, alcoholic drinks, side items, or desserts, that the cost of a simple seafood entrée and a vegetable on the side is reasonable! Maybe the reason rich people seem to be skinny is because they don't order appetizers, desserts, drinks, and sides, and maybe that's why skinny people seem to be rich too! Or, maybe not.

Either way….because of this, I found I was able to choose restaurants I normally wouldn't have gone to, and it made dining a lot more fun! Without much extra cost, you may find you get the benefit of giving yourself this

wonderful experience to look forward to. You'll be able to
spend all day or week looking forward to having a fantastic
meal prepared by a chef who really knows what he or she
is doing with food. Even if you've eaten your own grilled
Mahi-Mahi all week, you're going to eat a Mahi-Mahi like
you've never had in your life if you go to the right restaurant! The same goes for vegetables.

Great restaurants will let you make requests you
couldn't make at other restaurants. They'll grill a fish for
you and steam some asparagus for you, even if it's not on
the menu. They'll understand your dietary requests and go
out of their way to make you a great piece of fish, steak,
or chicken, and a great vegetable that you'll enjoy, because
you're paying them to do it. They'll take pride in making
you an awesome meal, and you'll enjoy every bite.

While on vacation in San Diego during Phase 2, we
went to a restaurant called Peohe's in Coronado. I was really
looking forward to it. I ordered an artichoke appetizer that
was literally just a whole artichoke, grilled. Eating just the
bits of "meat" off of that vegetable was one of the tastiest
things I've had in my life. It blew my mind, it was healthy
as anything, and I wasn't cheating! It was a great date night
while on vacation, yet I wasn't blowing it by eating some
huge portion of food.

This is a good time to mention that Derrick also likes
fancy restaurants. Derrick loves the way that steaks at nice
steakhouses are prepared. He likes how they bubble and
pop and he'll sometimes head out and pay way, *way* too
much for a nice dinner.

Eric found a way that Derrick could have his good
steaks, without paying so much for them. To do this, Eric

bought a cast iron skillet, and learned how to make a steak pop and bubble just like it does at a fancy restaurant, using his own oven at home. Then, Eric went out and bought a lot of Ziploc bags and really high-quality steaks and froze each steak individually. Then, Eric started to leave just enough steaks thawing in the 'fridge so that any time Derrick wants one, he can cook it and make it pop and sizzle just like a restaurant would within about 15 minutes! By doing this, Eric not only saved himself money, but he made steak days a lot easier.

By the way, Derrick also orders really great wines with those steaks, so Eric makes sure to keep the at-home bar stocked with the exact same selection, just 75 percent less expensive because it was bought at the grocery store!

It's probably best to stick with the advice of your nutritionist, which will most likely be to stay home and cook for yourself. However, if you find yourself stuck out and about, with no way to cook, great restaurants can help you, if they're visited in moderation, on this plan.

MY WEIGHT LOSS SAVIORS: LETTUCE WRAPS AND OMELETS

I'VE MENTIONED LETTUCE WRAPS many times throughout the book. It would be neglectful for me not to include them as one of my "weight loss saviors." I have to credit a friend at work for this idea. I was eating my own ground turkey and pepper mix with a fork at work when he spoke up and said, "why don't you bring in some lettuce and use it for lettuce wraps? Just chop the end off of a head of iceberg and the lettuce wraps peel right off."

Brilliant.

This is a very inexpensive, extra-healthy way to add a little texture and taco-ness to your mix.

Now, I make lettuce wraps all the time by creating a big mixture of protein and vegetables with seasoning. I bring it to work in a big container, and I make the lettuce wraps right there on my desk.

I can hide *all sorts* of vegetables from myself in these wraps! I'll often add chopped-up broccoli, zucchini, and squash, and I don't even know it's there when I'm eating it!

How many people do you know who eat two to three zucchinis and squashes per week, along with literally dozens of peppers, tomatoes, onions, and mushrooms? This really is a typical weekly intake for me. I'm constantly chopping vegetables with my Vidalia Chop Wizard (see the section about this under HCG Tools!). I'm eating great-tasting foods that I love, and they just happen to contain a ton of vegetables. You'd be surprised how many people at work ask what I'm making as I warm up my lunch in the storage container! They're jealous of my food, yet my food is the "diet food"!

To make lettuce wraps the way I do:

1) Mix up browned ground turkey with chopped peppers, onions, mushrooms, tomatoes, little hidden doses of squash, zucchini, and broccoli.

2) Cook them in a big saucepan with some no-sugar seasoning. (Choose any kind you like from the grocery store – experiment! I like just about any Mexican seasoning, like the kind used for burritos.)

3) Cut the bottom off of a head of iceberg lettuce, and then peel off pieces of lettuce that you can use to wrap up the Mexican mix.

I make a *huge* portion of the filler, and I separate it between containers, so that I can feed myself for days off of one cooking session.

I also found through this process that almost the same veggies can be used to make omelets. Omelets, along with lettuce wraps, became my new best friends. They get protein into you via eggs, and you can pack them with vegetables. You can easily transport them to work, or anywhere else you need to eat. If your nutritionist allows it, plan to eat a lot of these, especially if you want to get a lot of veggies into you, and your preference is not to eat whole vegetables or salads! You can use the same techniques you used to prepare vegetables for your wraps. Just cook up some eggs and dump the veggies in! Enjoy!

MY WEIGHT LOSS SAVIORS: THE BIGGEST LOSER

ONE OF THE THINGS that got me through this was *The Biggest Loser*. If you haven't seen this show, start watching it. Many seasons are available on iTunes and on DVD. The seasons contain tons of content, so I believe they're worth every penny you pay for them.

The Biggest Loser is a TV show on which people who need to lose a lot of weight (some lose hundreds of pounds) go to a ranch in California for months and months, where they work out daily with world-class trainers and eat healthy foods.

Let me just say that these people are my heroes. They got me through my weight loss, and I'm very thankful for their example. They inspired me. I downloaded seasons 11 through 15 on iTunes, and every day as I prepared my foods at 4:40 A.M., I'd watch *The Biggest Loser*.

Every day when I got home from work and couldn't drink alcohol with my friends like before, I'd watch that show. They made me realize that I was doing the right thing. They made me understand the path I was going down. They helped with a wealth of tips on what to eat and how to be healthier. The trainers are insightful and inspiring. The contestants start out in rough shape, with low confidence levels and little willpower. They end their time at the ranch as people who are driven, powerful, and inspiring. They "reset" their whole lives, and it's incredible to watch this happening.

I consider these people to be celebrities! I'd honestly be more star-struck meeting Danni Allen (a season 14 contestant) than I would by meeting Scott Baio right now. Okay maybe that's not the best example. But I'm not even kidding. As corny as this sounds, I feel like I went through their journey with them. As they were suffering and training hard, I was chopping vegetables and sticking to my plan. What I went through wasn't nearly as difficult or as long as the journey they went through, but without watching them all the time, I wouldn't have had the virtual "partner" I had by seeing their struggles and transformations.

I was insanely lucky to be able to meet contestants Dan Evans and Jackson Carter when I went to register for my half-marathon. Those guys probably hadn't met a fan as star-struck as me yet. As embarrassing as that might be for me to admit, I still stand by the fact that those contestants are heroes. They made massive changes in their habits and in their lives. While doing so, they inspired me and they helped me get through a tough period of time, and I'm thankful to them.

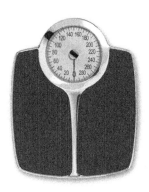

PART 7:
MY WEIGHT LOSS TOOLS

THERE ARE SOME FANTASTIC tools that helped me with my transformation, and I believe these can help you, as well. My hope is that these tools can help you to better align your habits with the advice you get from your doctor or nutritionist. They certainly did for me!

WEIGHT LOSS TOOLS:
MY WALL CHART

"We are what we repeatedly do. Excellence, then, is not an act, but a habit." –Aristotle

IN A SPONTANEOUS INTERVIEW with Brad Isaac, Jerry Seinfeld revealed a tip he had for young comics. Jerry said that the best way to be a better comic was to create better jokes and the way to create better jokes was to write every day. Seinfeld advised that young comics should get a big wall calendar and hang it on a "prominent wall." He said that for each day of comedy writing, he would put a red X on the calendar. Then, the objective was to just not break the chain of X's.[73]

This makes sense, doesn't it? As Aristotle said, "We are what we repeatedly do." What do comedians do? They write comedy. What do fit people do every day? They do fit things, like eat right and lose weight. The more we do this, the more we lose weight. So, if we should be tracking anything, it's our repetition of doing the right thing. I did this (and still do this) using big wall posters.

A friend of mine (brilliant guy) is a big believer in visual reminders. This guy is the opposite of "paperless." He likes paper, because he likes the act of writing something down, turning it into a physical artifact, and he likes that once it's written down, he can post it in very visible places where it's out in the open, as a reminder of what he's trying to do.

While I used to be someone who would try to file and organize everything, he reminded me that sometimes a huge, sticky-note type of pad taped to your wall will have a much bigger effect than a tiny electronic note filed away and "tagged." Big, three-foot-tall sticky notes on the wall are a tangible, ever-present reminder of what to do right. I took his advice and started using these huge wall notes at work. Then I ended up taking one home and using it to track my weight loss.

I've now used this technique to track my progress toward many goals over the years, and it was indispensable in this transformation process. Once you get over the initial explanation to visitors to your house and stop caring about what people think this will be a huge help to you.

My chart could be described as a giant calendar. Thinking about it now, you actually could use a calendar. The only reason I don't is that I get to customize the size of my boxes and I get to fit a lot of months onto one chart, without the white space between months.

I created my chart by dividing a poster board into weeks, with each week spanning a full row from left to right on the poster-board, and about 8-12 weeks represented from top to bottom.

You can use the big Post-It notes or just buy a grocery store poster board in the arts and crafts section like you would for your kid's school project. Grocery store clerks are always asking me why I'm buying these and, so far, I've amused myself with explanations like, "School project - my dad owns a hotel company and if I can pass all 12 grades I get to take over as CEO."

So I divide the poster boards into weeks and fit about eight weeks on each one. I set goals and use my markers to write on the poster board. It hangs right above my scale in the bathroom. I draw stupid little pictures that represent each goal, like a Christmas tree for Christmas, or a cruise ship for our cruise vacation. I do this because it very visibly and prominently reminds me of how many days I have until a big milestone is coming up. It's amazing – once you actually see a physical representation of the number of days to a major goal, you realize how short time is, and actually how long time is. It gives you great perspective.

During my transformation, I couldn't wait to fly home to see my family for Christmas, looking thin and in shape. It was just a goal of mine. Every Christmas (which is also my birthday), I always reflect on my goals, and do a lot of writing about where I'd like to be at the end of the coming year. I knew that this year, I'd feel a lot better about life if I drew that Christmas tree, put a goal weight under it, and worked toward that goal relentlessly. It worked. I felt great when I went home. I reached my goal!

There's something about this wall chart that just works for me. I'm a computer geek, and I've made many electronic to-do lists and spreadsheets, but none of them have been as effective for me as this graphical wall chart. I still track things electronically using spreadsheets, but I don't think I'll ever give up the use of this visual reminder of my goals and progress. With this chart on my wall, I seem to just "get it."

The same friend who introduced me to this added advice about it more recently. We were discussing how to track the progress of people working in an office, and he uses the same type of wall board for this. Someone had suggested that he replace the wall boards with electronic boards, which would automatically track progress. He laughed and let the person know that he just didn't get it. It wasn't about just the visual goals and progress on the wall, it was about the ritual of walking up and marking your progress. Just the act of grabbing the marker and writing down something you'd done was more important than the accuracy of what was written over the long term. You will find that you will look forward to this morning ritual, as you weigh in (hopefully very early!) and take a marker to a new day's box.

So, go out, get your big poster board and a bunch of colored markers, and have some fun with this. Don't try to make it perfect. The lines don't need to be straight, and the text doesn't need to look right to anyone but you. Write your goals on it. Is it another belt notch? A trip to the beach? A new outfit you get to buy? A special trip with the wife, husband, or kids? Visualize it and try your best to draw icons of it with the markers.

I also recommend that you consider using this for all of your goals, not just the weight loss transformation related goals. I use little drawings and markings on my chart to plan for a variety of goals and events, including financial

savings goals, visualizing the time I have to prepare for upcoming live music performances, planning for graduation
from my graduate program, and even writing and revising
this book!

WEIGHT LOSS TOOLS: MY SPREADSHEET: GOALS, LANDMARKS MILESTONES, REWARDS

THE POSTER BOARD MENTIONED above is a fantastic way to track your progress, but it has its limitations. Though it can give you a vivid visual reminder of your daily progress, it can't do calculations for you, and your writing real estate is limited. To get more specific and analytical with your goal tracking, I recommend using a spreadsheet.

As I've mentioned, I had very real, tangible goals while on this plan. At the beginning, I made a spreadsheet that included my daily goals and "milestone" goals, with descriptions of the feelings I'd have while reaching those goals. I kept close track of my progress, the original goals, and updated "realistic" targets that would change daily as my actual results changed. This set of goals was the same set that was on my wall chart, but more detailed.

I included planned rewards on this spreadsheet as well. One example was the watch I would buy once I got to my goal weight. Other planned rewards on the sheet included being able to fit into certain pairs of jeans again, or being able to wear a certain jacket I hadn't worn in years. Also, at the time, we had a company holiday party coming up and I knew that I'd weigh less for that and would fit into a suit. I knew that three years prior, I'd felt healthy at our holiday party and my suit fit right. I knew that if I hit my goal this time, that I'd be able to wear my suit and not have my belly busting out of it. That was a real treat.

One of the most helpful things about this sheet was when I did some research and tried to find, in my past, the times when I weighed different amounts. For example, I found that if I lost about 25 pounds, I would be exactly the weight I was the last time I fit into my suit correctly. I knew that because years prior to my weight loss, I had been recording my weight for some training I was doing for mountain climbing. I looked back at all of my old journals, spreadsheets, and even old wall charts I once had, to see where I was at different times in my life. From this, I was able to piece together a set of goals that was very informative. For example, "when you get to this weight, you'll be the same size you were in your sophomore year of college!" These motivated me to continue forward. I really enjoyed it when I'd get to a certain weight, knowing I was lighter than at a time I once felt very light!

One landmark that was very interesting to hit was when I was the exact same weight I was when I climbed Mt. Rainier in 2005. I have a picture of that climb above my desk, and people often used to ask me if that's really what I looked like! I felt like it was still "me," but obviously it was not. I now look like I did in the picture again!

I encourage you strongly to keep a detailed spreadsheet that includes daily tracking of your past, current, and future weight.

Use the spreadsheet daily, and let it be a visual guide so that you can see how many days you have before you hit a goal weight. Next to the goal weight, write some specifics about how you'll feel or what you'll look like when you reach that goal.

You should also use the spreadsheet to look back and track your weight through the past weeks, so you can see what your daily losses were, what your average losses were, and you can better predict your glide path toward future losses.

There's no specific or "right" way to make this spreadsheet. Just open up your spreadsheet application on your PC or Mac and get at it! If you've never done it before, you can quickly learn, just by messing around and typing in cells. I used Microsoft Excel, but if you don't have a license for Microsoft Office, you can use an online application like SmartSheet.[74]

WEIGHT LOSS TOOLS: VIDALIA CHOP WIZARD

ONE TOOL THAT HAS made my life much easier is my Vidalia Chop Wizard[75]. It's a tool that helps you to chop vegetables into small squares very quickly, and I owe a lot of my vegetable eating to this device. You simply put vegetables into it and crush them over a grid of blades by pressing down on the top, and you immediately have diced anything.

I use this to chop vegetables for my lettuce wraps, omelets, and pizzas. I literally use this on a daily basis! Sometimes I'll chop up vegetables, add seasoning and some ground turkey, and make my own type of "hamburger helper" that can just be eaten with a fork.

Regardless of how you use this, you'll find that you have a lot of vegetables to get into your stomach, and mixing them with seasonings and other various foods can help tremendously. I recommend buying one of these. It's extremely easy to clean. You can assemble it and disassemble it quickly. I leave it right on the counter, and it's probably my most-used piece of kitchen equipment other than a cutting board.

When vegetables go through the Vidalia Chop Wizard, they know they are close to being eaten by Eric.

WEIGHT LOSS TOOLS:
THE VEGGIE TO SPAGHETTI
CONVERTER

THE GEFU SPIRELLI SPIRAL Slicer is amazing.[76]

I bought a spiral slicer at Bed Bath and Beyond. It quickly cuts cylindrical-shaped vegetables like squash, zucchini, and carrots into ribbons that look like pasta noodles. This tool is incredibly good at its job.

Within minutes, you can turn a whole squash into a bowl of noodles, ready to be boiled in a pot just like ordinary spaghetti noodles (though they soften more quickly!), drain them, and serve them with pasta sauce over them.

This has become one of my favorite meals. I can literally eat a *pile* of squash – which is packed with nutrients and low in calories, with just a little low-sugar sauce and browned ground turkey, and be a very satisfied eater! This food gets even better when you store it in a container in the refrigerator overnight and eat it like "leftover spaghetti." The leftovers taste even more like leftover spaghetti than the fresh stuff tasted like fresh spaghetti! Just writing about this gets me excited.

Think about this: I am a guy who used to go out and eat a huge pile of spaghetti at a restaurant after work. Now,

I'm a guy who goes home and devours five whole squash. Five. It would be funny to see me go home and eat five squash, whole, while they're still shaped like squash. I just used a tool to reshape mine into spaghetti. Same vegetable, different shape. Also, while five may seem like a lot, you'd be surprised to see how my five-squash spaghetti pile is the same size spaghetti pile you'd get at your favorite Italian restaurant. In reality, I have gone home, eaten five whole vegetables, and gone to bed without getting hungry or craving any other foods! That's amazing, isn't it?

There's another dish out there called "spaghetti squash," which is actually a type of squash that, if cooked a certain way, can be broken down into strands. To me, this looks complex and time-consuming. The process above, using the spiral slicer, turns anything shaped like a cylinder into healthy pasta-shaped noodles, so it's a bit different than the actual "spaghetti squash."

I recommend that you buy this. It's the most fun an adult can have without actually breaking out the Play-Doh barbershop, and it can create quick, ultra-healthy meals for you and your family.

To make a good-sized bowl of pasta, it will take about three to four small squash, so you're going to need about twelve to sixteen to feed a family of four. You're going to look like you have some heavy squash greed at the grocery store, but just get used to it. Most people don't eat enough vegetables, and you can be proud to be feeding yourself and your family nutrient-dense foods, while others are shopping in the pasta aisle, picking up some simple starches for the gang at home. Enjoy!

WEIGHT LOSS TOOLS: SCALE AND TRACKING APPS

WHEN I FIRST STARTED my transformation, I was using an old scale that only weighed me in half-pound increments. This was both good and bad. It was good, because I didn't need to lose as much to make it seem like I was down a half-pound. It was bad, because I didn't need to gain as much to make it seem like I was up a half-pound! Regardless of whether either direction was good or bad, I came to the conclusion that I would rather have highly accurate weigh-ins than weigh-ins that made me feel good or bad. I wanted the truth, to the tenth of a pound, and I wanted it daily.

The scale I decided to go with, which I now ride daily, is the Smart Body Analyzer by Withings.[77] I love this scale for four reasons.

First, it syncs wirelessly with my iPhone through my home wireless network, so all I need to do is weigh in, and my weight and body fat percentage show up in my Withings app.

Second, it weighs accurately to the tenth of a pound, meaning that the slightest fluctuation in my weight is recorded. This helps because I like to really be accurate about my correction days or "steak days." When I go anywhere above two pounds above my LIW, I'm immediately going to do a correction day, and since my scale doesn't round at all, I know when this happens and I correct it.

The third reason I love the scale is that the app that goes along with it is extremely passive aggressive. It says things like, "We lost 3 pounds this week, let's not lose sight of our goal." I love a scale that insults you even when you kept pretty close to your goal weight in a maintenance phase.

The fourth and final reason I love this scale is that, for a full-size deal, it's somewhat portable. I brought it with me on the cruise and on a family vacation to Wisconsin. It's not the lightest thing to add to your suitcase, but it's reasonably light, considering you get a full-size bathroom scale to travel with.

Along with the Withings app that my scale syncs to automatically, I also sync that app with yet *another* weight tracking app that gives me all sorts of views of my progress. This app is called Monitor Your Weight.[78] Using this app is easy, because it imports data right from the Withings app. You can also use it without the Withings app, by just entering your weight manually.

The strength of the Monitor Your Weight app is that it offers multiple views that are very useful. One of my favorites is the "monthly" view, which shows a calendar view of your weigh-ins. I find that my weight fluctuates through the week, but that those fluctuations are very consistent when observed week-over-week. For example, on Thursdays I'm my lightest, because Monday through Thursday are my most regimented, disciplined days while I'm at work. I find that over the weekends, as hard as I try, I just don't get enough water through my system like I do on weekdays, and I end up putting on a little extra weight (within one to two pounds usually) due to that. Using the "monthly" view in this app, it's very easy for me to compare Mondays to other Mondays, as opposed to comparing a Monday to a Thursday, as I might with a straight-line tracking system. If I weigh one to two pounds less on a Sunday than I did the previous Sunday, I know I'm doing very well, and I'm set up for a great week at work, where I can possibly lose another two to three pounds easily. If I'm up a bit on a Monday compared to the last Friday, I can look at the last Monday to see if that was abnormal. I think it's important for you to take regular patterns like this into account as you monitor your weight, so that you don't get discouraged every Sunday (or whichever day your high weigh-ins may tend to be), and you don't get overly happy every Thursday (or whichever day your low weigh-ins may tend to be). Businesses use the same method when tracking their performance. A toy store certainly wouldn't compare the Christmas shopping months to February or March, and they also wouldn't compare a big shopping day like Saturday to a workday like Tuesday. If you find that your weight gains and losses are cyclical in the way that mine are, try using this app to help you take this approach!

Once you get these apps set up, and if you decide to spend a little extra money on the Withings (or any other wireless scale) you can stand on your scale and just look at your phone. All of your weight measurements will be right there on the screen, with no data-entry required. My morning ritual is to get up, weigh in, write on the wall chart with my marker, and then not have to record anything else, knowing that my data is stored in the phone already.

Research actually shows that apps such as the Withings app and the Monitor Your Weight app can aid in weight loss when used in conjunction with weight loss programs, especially for tech-savvy users.[79] I suggest checking into these to aid your progress!

WEIGHT LOSS TOOLS: CLEAR, AND TO DO LISTS

ONE OF THE THINGS that really helped me out on this journey was an app for the iPhone called Clear.[80] Clear is a to-do list app that syncs lists between your Mac, iPhone, iPad, or any device you have in the Apple family. There are probably apps like this for other devices. This is just the one I used. You can also use a notecard to do what I did with it.

There are two lists that I made that really guided my day. I still use both lists every day. The first list is a list of water that I have taken in daily. It's simply a numbered list, going from one to eight. Each time I drink a full bottle of water, I mark it as "complete" on the list. The Clear app allows me to then go back and mark them as incomplete the next morning, so that I can reuse the same list daily without much extra effort.

I like Clear because it's simple, it's easy to use, and it does *no more than exactly what you need it to do*. Complexity for no reason can create hassle. Clear has simplified the to-do list. I found this to be a perfect, sustainable way to track my food and water intake, and I continue to use it to this

day. I think the people at realmacsoftware.com have created a great, efficient app that's handy for tracking things,
and I wish them continued success.

WEIGHT LOSS TOOLS: MY JOURNAL

RESEARCH PUBLISHED IN THE *International Journal of Behavioral Nutrition And Physical Activity* suggests that keeping a diary has been empirically proven to help boost weight loss effort, so it comes as no surprise that my nutritionist encouraged me to keep a journal.[81] I did just that, and it became so fulfilling and rewarding to me, that the journal grew into this book.

The journal is important because it holds you accountable daily to doing the right things. When you do the right things, it makes you happy to write them in the journal. When you mess up a bit, you hold yourself accountable by writing it down. You also tend to forgive yourself more quickly when you write something down. You put it on paper, and then it's behind you. Research published in *Psychology and Health* suggested that mindfulness and self-compassion mediated avoidance and negative thoughts with weight loss and that keeping a diary (or journal) increased mindfulness and self-compassion, decreased negative thoughts, and supported weight loss significantly.[82]

I personally found writing daily about my goals and my progress to be energizing and cathartic. It became very fun to look back at the journal entries about my belt notches, my new clothes, and even at the beginning about the rash on my belly being annoying. It's still fun to look at, and it's become the basis for this very book.

The journal ended up being so useful for me that I now write a daily journal including every area in which I'm trying to progress. I include a daily column about my master's degree, my music performance and composition, my writing of this book, my nutrition and weight, my marathon training, my financial planning and investing, my relationships, my general notes, and even my specific examples of overcoming temptation. I record my feelings and progress daily because it holds me accountable and keeps me in check in every area. I look forward to getting up early and writing about the previous day. I also have something to look back on to see where I was doing well and where I messed up in each area. Even better, as evidenced by this book, these journals have become so robust that they can sometimes turn into something bigger. Who knows what's next after this book? It could be one on personal finance, or on leadership! I look forward to continuing to write about these areas to see what becomes valuable for others.

I think that, no matter how big or small you decide to make the effort, you should keep a journal of your progress on this plan. Even if your progress is terrible, write about it. If you're happy about something, write about it. If you

messed up and you're upset and you need to forgive yourself, write about it. The accumulation of these writings will
help you more than you think, and the act of writing is in
and of itself, a true blessing.

WEIGHT LOSS TOOLS:
ONLINE RESOURCES

THERE ARE SO MANY wonderful resources online that can help you as you progress. Use them! All it takes is a Google search when you have a question about weight loss, nutrition, or HCG, and you'll find hundreds of helpful communities, recipes, tools, and calculators. There are many people out there going through what you're going through, and they're willing to connect with you and help you. Remember, you should first trust the information given to you by your doctor and nutritionist. Then, when you need a little extra guidance late at night, on a weekend, or just with something small like how to make a specific recipe, you can find almost everything you need right online. Take some time to search online communities for HCG information, and check out the helpful videos on YouTube, as well. Resources and support are everywhere around you!

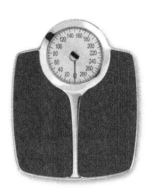

PART 8:
A LITTLE PHILOSOPHY

ALL OF THIS ADVICE is intended to help you achieve your goals. Now, let's take some time to discuss mindset, psychology, and the belief systems that can help you get there and cause others to influence you to fail, if you're not careful!

WHY PEOPLE WANT
YOU TO FAIL

"It is often the case that you have to fire certain friends or retire from particular social circles to have the life you want." -Tim Ferriss, The 4-Hour Workweek[83]

ONE OF THE THINGS you'll find when you set out to do anything great in life, including losing weight, is that people around you will say negative things about it. This comes in many forms, ranging from the blatant "That won't work," to a more masked, "How are you going to manage that with everything you have going on?" It's sad, but a lot of people, knowingly or unknowingly, will actually want you to fail. These people may even include your family, your spouse, and your closest friends.

I'm fortunate that I have had a few people in my life who have always been positive toward any goal I set out to attain. My father, my mother, and my sister, no matter what I tell them I'll do, always reply, "You *should* do that, you'd be great at it!" My aunts, uncles, cousins, and grandparents have always been the same way. I'm forever thankful for that and I also realize that not everyone has that type of support around them.

When you're trying to accomplish a goal like this, you need to seek out that type of support. More importantly, and on the other side of that coin, you need to rid your life of the people around you who tell you you'll fail. You need to stay away from them, and if you must be around them for short periods of time, you need to laugh it off and stay strong around them.

There are some people out there on downward spirals trying (sometimes unintentionally) to wreck their lives for whatever reason. They're everywhere, and just like a drowning person who is reaching for anything that floats can drown a lifeguard, your friend can also drown you by including you in her bad habits. You can't let that happen. You need to take a hard look at who around you influences you to do things you don't really care to do, and you need to say goodbye or stay away from them, even if it's just until you're well into Phase 4.

If you remember the story of Commodore Longfellow that I told earlier in the book, you'll recall that I made sure the Commodore was going to be out of town for a few critical weeks during the beginning of my transformation. Commodore Longfellow certainly is not a bad influence in all aspects. I look up to the Commodore in many ways, it's just that healthy eating is not one. In this case, I just made sure to stay away from the Commodore long enough to transform my habits to the point that I could be strong enough around him to start associating again. You'll need to decide whether or not the people around you who have a negative influence on your eating habits (or other habits you're trying to change) are going to need to stay out of the picture until you've grown stronger, or whether they'll be out of the picture for good. If it's the former, you may be able to help them to change when you start hanging out again. If it's the latter, it may be a tough decision for you, but sometimes this kind of strength is necessary when you want to make positive changes to the way you live your life.

Also, I would be doing an injustice without saying this: it's okay, once you've established new habits, to go back and associate with these folks if your intention is to help them, and you believe they can be helped. However, don't go back too soon. If you've ever flown on a plane, you've heard again and again during the safety drill that you need to put *your* air mask on before you put your child's air mask on. The reason? You won't be much help to anyone, including that child if you've already passed out! The case is the same here. You won't be much good to your friends if they suck you back into the habits that got you into rough shape in the first place.

Take the time to truly help yourself and establish new habits. Then, and only then, can you return to try to help anyone (if they even want your help). I still am very careful about re-entering some of my old circles, or, if I do re-enter, about staying there for more than an hour or so. Helping people is important, and I encourage you to do it, but only once you've taken the time to really help yourself.

People who are bad influences also tend to put themselves in situations that can be negatively influential. Make sure to stay out of situations where these types of people will be doing things that are counterproductive to your goals. If these people are having a pizza party, do not go. If these people are eating a birthday cake at work, do not go to the sing-along. These people will absolutely tell you you're a downer for not going. Forget them. They're the downer, all pudgy and sluggish, eating cake and pizza, and drinking a soda in the middle of the workday like it's normal. Get away from these people. If you need to, be very direct and tell them you're making decisions to make your life better, and that you're done with that kind of eating, period.

People get uncomfortable when you break away from the patterns of failure that they live every day. People don't like it when you stop doing the bad things they're doing, like overspending, drinking too much, or taking smoke breaks. Think about how much people try to convince you to eat a piece of cake when they're having one. Think about how awkward they try to make you feel just over a piece of birthday cake! Think about how much people try to convince you to stay at a party or at a bar where everyone is drinking the night away, when you tell them you're going to leave early. They don't want you to leave, because if you leave, they're the ones wasting their lives all the sudden. Before someone stands up and says, "I can't waste any more of my life here," everyone else has no benchmark. When someone says, "I'm going to be different," and others know she's right, things are going to feel really awkward. Get comfortable with that awkwardness. You don't need to fix everyone, but you do need to remove yourself.

People who seem to be your dear friends are sometimes your friends because you're both carrying out the same poor habits. Misery loves company. If they don't want to come along with you for the ride as you improve (or at least support you wholeheartedly and genuinely), you may very well need to let them go. That may be the price of change, in this case, and you need to be willing to pay it. Are you?

LIMITING BELIEFS

SOMETHING I THINK WE need to discuss in order for you to be in the right frame of mind during your transformation is the idea of "limiting beliefs."

There's a story I love to tell about limiting beliefs. A grown elephant is standing in place, tied by a length of rope to a small stake that's stuck in the ground. Though the elephant could easily walk in any direction and pop the stake right out, she never tries. The reason is that from the time the elephant was a little baby elephant, her trainers had kept her tied to the same stake with the same length of rope. Sure, the baby elephant had tried to pull out the stake, but it didn't work. After a while, the elephant accepted that she was stuck next to the stake, and, regardless of her true ability, she stopped trying to pull it out.

Limiting beliefs are those beliefs that limit you from trying things because you think they are impossible. People often form these types of beliefs because of something they tried and failed at (like the elephant), something they read, or something somebody told them. To give you a simple example, if you absolutely believed that it was impossible to consistently lose more than two pounds per week, you would probably never try to lose more than two pounds per week. You would know that was impossible, so why would you try? This happened to be one of my limiting beliefs, before I discovered this plan and shattered the belief entirely.

Think about all the "beliefs" you have. Think about all the hard lines you put in place that you can't cross. We get all of this information accumulated in our heads about what is and what is not possible, and then we limit ourselves!

I read a daily newsletter about finance, and in it, there was a column that blew my mind. One of the articles said that the FTC published a list of things about weight loss that are "never true." One of the things listed as a claim that is never true was, "You can lose more than three pounds a week for more than four weeks – and do it safely, with no potential ill effects to your health."

Yet, how many times have we seen *The Biggest Loser* contestants defy that? They do it every single week, every single season. They're working out, eating right, losing weight, and having tremendous medical progress, yet here we have an article telling a general population that it's impossible!

The danger here is that people will read this, without knowing differently, and they'll believe that fast weight loss is impossible. This may cause them to slow their own progress or, worse, to give up altogether!

The bigger problem here is that in many areas of life, we create limiting beliefs.

Think about some of the great things that have been accomplished in the world. The cure of polio. Putting a man on the moon. Any successful venture starts with something seemingly impossible, yet all of a sudden it becomes possible because people have a vision and simply begin to believe it is possible. Are your limiting beliefs holding you back from great discoveries about how to improve your health or your life? Identify them, and bust the myths that are holding you back!

I highly recommend identifying your own limiting beliefs. Again, know thyself. Realize what you've gone around believing for years, and challenge, or at least verify those beliefs. Don't let yourself be tricked into mediocrity by believing something is impossible when it is, in fact, very possible! Go see your doctor. Get good advice. Seek out a nutritionist. Decide what you are able to lose safely. Then, once you have this advice on paper, act like a horse with blinders on and follow that plan perfectly!

"HEALTHY" FOODS AND THE NEED FOR A PLAN

SINCE WE'VE COME THIS far, I'd like to talk to you about something that can easily get on all of our nerves, which is the topic of "healthy foods." Somewhere along the way, people started to refer to individual foods as "healthy" and "unhealthy." As I was mid-transformation and following my plan, people would say things to me like, "You can have whole grains, right? Whole grains are healthy, why can't you have these crackers?"

I always get irritated when I read a Men's Health magazine and it talks about "the one food that helps you have a smaller belly." Foods don't give you a smaller belly on their own. There is no miracle food. You need a PLAN, not a one-food article.

Likewise, when someone offers me a piece of chicken and says, "Why can't you have this? This is chicken, this is healthy," I'll admit, I kind of want to punch them.

People just don't understand. Though some foods are very nutrient-dense and other foods are not as nutrient-dense, it's all about planning and eating the right things *as part of a comprehensive plan*. There is no one good food or one bad food you can just eat on its own. People need a plan for each day that gets them all of the nutrients they need. Kale may be "healthy," but you can't *just* eat that! Everything fits as part of a balanced diet. The reason I wouldn't take the chicken from my friend isn't because it was *bad* for me on its own, it's because I'd already planned out my day, and that chicken wasn't a part of the plan. I wasn't willing to divert from a well-balanced and tasty plan just to eat that chicken, and therefore I didn't take it. The same reason he was confused is the reason he seems to maintain his current physical state. He's evaluating each piece of food he puts in his mouth, without thinking about the big picture. Though he may choose the "healthy" ones, he has no comprehensive plan, no goal, and no accountability. In the end, the big picture is what really counts. Don't judge foods. Make a full plan that includes a variety of foods that, all together, complete your nutrition picture.

In the same mindset, don't judge foods as "healthy" and just start eating them if they're not on your plan. If they're not on the plan, they're not on the plan. Don't eat them. I know a guy who "tried" HCG and wasn't losing weight. I asked him what he was eating, and he said, "I eat a lot of almonds." "Almonds?" I asked him. "Who told you that you could have any almonds at all?"

He said, "Almonds are healthy, right?"

I said, "Almonds can be a part of a healthy diet if eaten in moderation, but they don't belong anywhere near you on HCG Phase 2 when you're cutting calories. Who told you to eat almonds?"

He replied, "I always eat a lot of almonds."

I took the time to show him what was on my plan, so that he could get an understanding of what a comprehensive plan looked like. Once he saw the plan, he actually realized the kind of commitment it would take, and shortly thereafter, he gave up. This wasn't a bad thing, it's just that he wasn't ready yet. He was thinking that if he just chose healthy foods, it would get him to his goal. He wasn't ready to follow a structured daily plan yet.

All food is part of a bigger plan. All foods are going to have some nutritional value, and some foods are more nutrient-dense than others. Some foods contain the nutrients you need for the day, and some foods you may not need to complete your plan for the day. Can olives be healthy? As part of a master plan, olives can have some good healthy fat in them. They can also be very high in sodium. Chicken, is that healthy? It can be a great source of protein, but you can't just eat chicken. You have to have a plan that includes a full day of good nutrition, and looking at each food as a "yes/no" isn't the way to do it. You need to look at the big picture of a day and decide how you're going to get the nutrients you need throughout the whole day. At some point, someone might catch you eating a saltine cracker and think, "That's a bad food." But you're eating four of them and you need that little boost of energy from the starch to help maintain your energy levels. It's not "bad" as part of a plan. So don't listen to people who ask, "Why aren't you eating this? This is healthy, right?" "You'll eat a saltine, but you won't eat my chicken? That's dumb."

Don't just think that because a food has been labeled as "healthy," it belongs in your mouth while you're following a plan. Get this plan from your nutritionist, then (surprise) follow the plan, follow the plan, follow the plan.

PRODUCTIVE ANXIETY

ONE OF THE ABSOLUTE blessings I got from my time with HCG was something I like to call "productive anxiety." You should look forward to having this!

I started to do so well with my weight loss that I actually looked forward to getting up early each morning. I'd bounce out of bed, I'd weigh in, I'd do some journaling, and I'd grab some coffee. I'd be ready to go for the day, long before anyone else was awake and even thinking of getting started.

Whereas before, I would have been working for my job and just trying to get through another day, I now felt like I was living life for me and my job was there for income. Even though I found my job to be challenging and I still cared very much about my organization's success, I now had other things I was inspired to do! Out of nowhere, I began to want to write more. I began to want to read more. That turned into something even bigger. I began to actually feel like I couldn't pack enough into each day! I began to think about all the books I wanted to read, the skills I wanted to learn, and the things I wanted to write and share with others. I actually began to have anxiety about not being productive enough! Whereas before, all of my anxiety was about whether or not I'd get to work on time and do the things I was supposed to there, that now became only a portion of what I wanted to accomplish, and I started to yearn for more. I started to make my life more significant. I started to think about the people I could help, the causes I could promote, and the impact I could make on the world. I called this feeling "productive anxiety."

All of this came from a simple, quick loss of 30 pounds. Just that 30 pounds of weight was holding me back from all of this. Now, as I wrap up the first book I'll publish, I realize that this wasn't about the weight as much as it was about changing my state of being and reaching a new level of consciousness. My health and low energy levels were holding me back from all this, and it's only just the beginning! I encourage you to start your journey ASAP, because it's not just about belt notches, it's about the person you get to become once those pounds are melted off.

Trust me, there are places in your life that lie just beyond the horizon – you just can't see them until you swim out there a little ways. The first 30 pounds I lost made a massive difference in the horizon my eyes were able to see. I believe that the same will be true for you, and that this effort is worthwhile for reasons far beyond the ones you will write down when you begin this journey.

ALCOHOL

AS I'VE MENTIONED, I'M a guy who enjoys having a drink from time to time. However, things have changed greatly about that. Almost every day after work, I used to head out with my buddies for a cocktail at happy hour. We'd head out of work after a long day, stressed and ready to talk even more about work – just in a different setting. My norm was to throw back a Tanqueray and tonic or two. I might have a Coors Light. At the time, I would actually look forward to that drink at the end of the day. I'd look forward to the strong taste of the gin and the way it quickly made the overwhelming stress-feeling disappear. Many of you can probably relate.

I tell you this now with complete honesty and sincerity. I absolutely no longer have that same want for alcohol. I can still drink, but I no longer look forward to it in that way. Moreover, it's difficult for me to decide on what kind of drink I might want, because I literally think about the taste of hard liquor and the first thing I associate it with is a poison taste. That may sound strange, but Strong drinks like gin just haven't been the same for me since completing Phase 2.

I relate this to the example of my uncle, who had heart surgery. After the surgery, inexplicably, my uncle said that even though he used to love to drink beer, he literally no longer had a taste for it. He just didn't want it or enjoy it. I'm the same now with any sort of hard liquor. The only thing I really enjoy now is red wine, and even that took some getting used to. I used to drink more beer, but these days it just feels like sugar and empty carbs to me, so I've given that up on most occasions as well. I'd rather drink San Pellegrino if I need something refreshing, and I just don't want to deal with the aftermath or weight gain from the beer.

Being honest, before HCG, I'd have at least one drink five to six nights per week. After HCG, I'm down to two to three nights at most. I just don't want the stuff like I used to. I have to thank my nutritionist and the HCG plan for that, because even though I never faced the consequences that some people do when they've had too many drinks, I'm think that in a matter of time, I might have. There have been too many mornings in my life when I've woken up in a haze because I had one too many the night before. Even just a few drinks can ruin the next morning. You may not wake up with a headache, but you certainly don't jump out of bed, grab a coffee, and continue writing your next book. I'm not sure if you can relate to this or not, but alcohol used to give me a physical feeling I'll compare to "guilt." Even if I hadn't done anything out of line with my values, I'd have the feeling that I just wasn't myself. I like living now without as much of it. I can't believe that in such a short time I lost a taste for it, and I'm very thankful to be drinking down a different path. I think that this was a great benefit of this plan, and I think that if you find yourself looking forward to that drink after work, you might also find that this plan helps you to change direction toward a more productive state.

TAKING GREAT CARE OF YOURSELF

THIS GOES ALONG WITH makeover week, as I mentioned above. It's strange, looking back, how much I had given up on my appearance. I didn't care what I wore or if my hair was cut or if I even shaved my face on any given day. I had given up on being able to be a healthy person, and I certainly had lost any interest in trying to look attractive. I put those thoughts in the back of my mind, like they didn't matter to me.

The thing is, even though I'd given up, these things *did* matter to me, and as I went through life pretending they didn't, I got sad. I was sad that my belt was cutting into my stomach. I was sad that my shirts didn't fit right. When I lost some weight, things got better, and I started to take even better care of myself.

In the two years leading up to this transformation, I would rarely have gone to a spa, gotten a massage, or thought to pick out clothes for a day that might make me look decent. Now, I'm more focused on taking care of myself. Part of it may be vanity, but to me, it's about feeling good and being confident. I'm not advising that you go out and buy clothes to impress people, or get massages you can't afford. I'm suggesting that as part of your transformation, you begin to focus on taking great, great care of yourself. Find a Groupon and get a massage. Find an affordable store you like and pick out some clothes that fit you better. Heck, get a spray tan if it makes you feel good! Start doing things that show pride in your body and your image, and it will begin a cycle that will cause you to continue to show pride in your body and image. This momentum can help your transformation to feel more rewarding and to speed you along on the right path.

GIVE YOURSELF HOPE

IT'S MY BELIEF THAT people need to have things to look forward to. I actually include these things in my journal. I like to ask people, "What are you looking forward to right now the most, in any area of your life? A vacation? An accomplishment? Reaching a goal? Seeing someone you know? A visit from a friend?"

If you have nothing to look forward to, life can get pretty bland. When I was a kid, I worried a lot. I wondered how my parents could be happy if they didn't have a summer break like I did from school. After all, that's all I'd look forward to! I now realize that I was right to worry. Adults often don't have enough to look forward to!

This also works on a small scale. Too often, people look forward to "treats" they give themselves through the day. They might look forward to that next smoke break, or that after-work cocktail. They might look forward to a big meal in the evening, or hitting up a fast food joint at lunch. Do you see a pattern here? We often reward ourselves with things that are bad for us. But it doesn't need to be this way! Replace these rewards with those that are healthy! Look forward to a low calorie cup of coffee! Look forward to that cold San Pellegrino! Look forward to some great stuffed peppers at lunch! Look forward just to seeing your kids after work, working on your garden, watching your favorite TV show, or taking a walk with your family after dinner. On weekends, look forward to taking a road trip to your favorite local destination or walking nine holes with a golf buddy! Let's replace the big restaurant meals you're looking forward to with activities that aren't counter to your new goals. Take some time to find out what you like to look forward to, and look forward to it!

Next, take an inventory of the big things you're looking forward to, possibly over the next year, or two, or three. What are you looking forward to? A promotion? A big purchase? A new car? A vacation for your family? A new addition to the house? A new addition to the family? Starting school after saving up enough tuition money? Graduating from school with a new degree? If you can't immediately come up with things like these to look forward to, I believe you need to *make* something! Write it down! Put it in your journal way up ahead on a given date, and strive toward it, whatever it is – the *more* you have to look forward to, the *better* life will be!

Once you have some things written down, make countdowns and track your progress toward those things. Without that, life has to be pretty sad. Without hope, there is no life, and there is no happiness. No matter what personally drives you, give yourself that hope.

ON PAYING ATTENTION
TO OUR THOUGHTS

DAVID ALLEN IS ONE of the leading writers on personal productivity. One thing I've learned from him recently is that we need to pay attention to the things that occupy our thoughts. In a recent book, David Allen shared that when he is working with clients, he asks them what they are giving their attention to.[84] In other words, what is taking up space in their mind – occupying their thoughts? This is important, because it allows David to help his clients to become more free to be in-the-moment, doing what matters most, instead of worried about various ideas, actions, or objects that are strewn about their offices and minds.

What are we giving attention to? It's important that we understand this at all times, so that we can better focus our attention and direction. Research published in the *Journal of Applied Psychology* shows that this concept of mindfulness, when practiced, may lead to an increase in psychological wellbeing, as well as life and job satisfaction. The same mindfulness can lead to decrease in stress levels and emotional exhaustion.[85]

Philosopher Ekhart Tolle wrote of a similar concept in his book, *The Power of Now: A Guide to Spiritual Enlightenment.* According to Tolle, we are not our thoughts. Your thoughts are not *you* but just something you happen to be occupied with! So, from a practical standpoint, **think about what you're thinking about!**

What are you giving attention to? You may find that a thought occupying your mind for minutes – even hours – is totally negative. When I focused on my own thoughts, it was amazing what kind of negativity still existed deep within me!

What if I never finish this book? What if I do finish it and nobody reads it? What if 30 pounds isn't significant enough for people to care about this advice?

When I realized these fears were nagging at me, I realized they were also holding me back. The reason I wasn't writing as fast as I wanted to was because I was scared of what would happen at the end. I was doubting myself. Once I realized it, this was powerful! I was able to understand what my thoughts were guiding me to do, and I was able to make adjustments to my nutrition, physiology, and state of mind in order to accomplish what I wanted to accomplish.

The same happens with weight loss. Be very aware of the doubts you are having, and then, realize they are just doubts, but don't need to be made real. What doubts are holding you back? Do you wonder if, once you lose the weight, you will still be able to enjoy the meals you do now with your overweight friends? Do you worry that you'll "gain it all back?" Why are you scared to do what you know will be healthy for you? It is critical that you get into your own mind, and clear these thoughts out, before they stop you from your ultimate progress!

Recognize what occupies your thoughts and attention, rationalize it, and put it behind you! You may be worried that once you succeed, you won't be able to continue your habits. So, deal with that when you come to it! Let "future you" figure all that out! For now, focus on losing that weight!

You may worry that you won't want to be "active" once you get skinnier. Don't worry about that! Heck, I'm healthy and I still don't like kayaking – too mundane for me. No worries. Just deal with it later. Put your mind to a goal – get healthy – fit into your old jeans – *then* go after bigger things. Recognize when you have thoughts of doubt, but let them be no more than thoughts, realize there's no evidence to back them, realize they don't have to be true, and *stay the course*. Don't let those thoughts destroy the actions you are taking!

MAKE THE BODY'S RESILIENCY WORK FOR YOU, INSTEAD OF AGAINST YOU

The body is resilient.

THE BODY IS RESILIENT in many ways. Knowing this and taking advantage of it can be a key to your weight loss and your maintenance of a successful weight for the rest of your life.

Think about it. If you needed to wake up tomorrow at the same time you wake up every day, would you really need an alarm clock? Even on days when you plan to sleep in, do you find your eyes tend to open right about the same time your alarm would usually go off? When you try to go to bed earlier than usual, do you have trouble falling asleep? What if you tried to eat a gigantic meal at a time of day when you never eat? Could you? It often takes a very deliberate and forced change to do anything differently than we normally do. It's like trying to get rid of jet lag. It's tough!

Your body wants to maintain its momentum – it wants to keep doing what it's been doing.

In my experience, it's the same with your body weight. Do you find you've been the same weight for a long time, gaining or losing only very slowly, no matter what you seem to do? I've found that when you get to a certain "set point," and you stay there for a very long time, it takes quite a shock to your body out of that point. This is bad in the beginning because it's tough to lose weight. But this is great in the end, because it's tough to gain weight once you've achieved a new set point!

I found later in Phase 4 that I was binging more than I should, but every time I binged or every time I did something dumb (like the time I ate a can of Spaghetti-Os after visiting a wine bar), I'd be right back on it the next day, and find that my weigh-ins were just fine! I wouldn't break out of my set point range because it was established. My advice is to use this to your advantage!

To do this, I think there are two things that can help you.

1) As I've mentioned many times already, get your body used to sleeping and eating at the right times so that you eventually become tired, awake, and hungry when you want to be tired, awake, and hungry.

2) At all costs, once you hit your last injection weight to begin Phase 3, stay there for as long as you possibly can. When I reached this weight, I immediately switched my written and recorded goals to focus on consistency, instead of weight loss. My goal became to spend as many consecutive days as possible within two pounds of my Last Injection Weight. I

would count the days on my wall chart and try to beat my record without exiting that weight range. It was like the signs at factories that say, "This many days without an accident." If I went 14 days without having to do a steak day, I'd then try to beat it by going 15 or more days the next time. Remember Seinfeld's calendar filled with weeks of red Xs. Make your goal about consistency. When you reach your weight loss goal, shift your focus to disciplined maintenance, and don't lose focus!

When you do this consistently, you'll find over time that a one-day mistake will rarely pull you out of your weight range. At first, your weight may bounce around, but after just a week or so of staying steady, it will take quite a shock to pull you out of that two-pound range. Just like on day three of vacation in a different time zone you start to lose your jet lag, on Day 3 or so of eating the wrong things and sleeping at the wrong times, it is enough to start to beat up your weight loss a bit. I suggest, for this reason, that you're very careful about giving yourself any sort of pattern-changing break on weekends, and I strongly suggest you limit vacations to shorter, three to four day lengths. If you must give yourself a break, do it for a day, not a weekend, and then get right back on that horse. If this happens for two days, get right back on that horse and even do a correction day if you need to. On day three, you may find yourself to be pretty out of whack. I learned this the hard way on my all-you-can-eat cruise, and it took me a couple of weeks to really get back into a steady, solid range of my LIW.

If you do find that you've broken your pattern for a number of days, I suggest that you get in to see your nutritionist as fast as you can. Do anything it takes. See a friend. Call your employee assistance plan at work! See a behavioral counselor! Whatever you need to do, do it to get back to consistency. It's easy to recover from a short lapse in judgment, and hard to recover from a multi-day pattern change. Finally, no matter what, realize it's never too late to turn it all back around. Remember the quote from the movie *Vanilla Sky*, "Every passing minute is another chance to turn it all around." Grab a bottle of water, grab some coffee, grab some fruit, and let's get back to work.

THE WORLD IS UPSIDE DOWN

IT GOES WITHOUT SAYING, but the world is upside down right now when it comes to health and nutrition. I'm not here to assign blame, but I want to share this observation with you.

People think eating unhealthy food all day is normal, and it's not okay.

Quite frankly, now that I've been through this, I can't really believe the stuff that goes on right in front of our faces. I wrote this section from a restaurant, while I watched a table of people order these burgers with huge, buttery buns. After the diet-change I had just been through, the food just looked disgusting to me. The group was eating these huge burgers, and these folks were already pretty overweight. Here's what I was thinking at the time.

The problem isn't that they're doing it – the problem is that it's *normal*. The problem is that I'm one of the only people in this room – probably *the* only person in this room, thinking all of this eating is crazy. The true craziness is that the norm has become the norm!

This is a typical Saturday evening for people! They go out, they order food that will kill them, and they eat it all. The norm is disgusting. It's like the movie *The Matrix*, where everyone is plugged into a battery somewhere, yet nobody seems to know or care. The wool is pulled over all of our eyes, and everyone seems to think it's normal to ingest sugary soda all day long or go to a gas station and order a huge slushee.

People think it's normal to go to a restaurant, order a huge burger with mayonnaise all over it, and eat the whole thing. Worse, when people do the opposite and go get good vegetables to cook, they're looked at as if they're the exception! Sitting at work, I watched a friend of mine get up, go to the vending machine, and grab some chips and a coke. Nobody thought anything of it! It has become normal to ingest sugary soda and snack foods all day long, every day! The *norm* is what is wrong. The fact that someone can be 40 pounds overweight and be seen as "normal" is insane. It shouldn't be normal but it is.

When your buddy decides to order a salad at lunch, and just have a tiny bit of dressing – *he's* looked at as the one that's on a "diet." It should be the opposite. Everyone who orders the insanely huge burger at an everyday lunch in the middle of a workday should be looked at as crazy. The guy with the salad should be yelling, "What are you guys doing – you have to be joking, right?" The whole world is headed for a train wreck and nobody is even tapping the brakes! It's like back when we were installing asbestos in every home in America, and nobody said a word, but it's worse, because we all *know* this stuff is poisonous! "Go ahead and just put that right in there, guys – it's in everyone else's house, so it may as well be in mine." It's like when we were bloodletting to cure disease, even after we found out that it didn't work! Rome is burning! We are going to die! Our kids are going to die!

The saddest part about it is this: The person in front of me taking a bite of that burger has hopes and dreams and is beautiful. I look at this woman with the burger and I wonder if when she sees herself in the mirror, whether or not she feels like this is how she wants to be. My guess is that she is somewhat like I was, feeling a bit trapped and limiting herself without even knowing the extent to which she is limited. If she's at all like I was, she's sad about who she has become, and even worse, she's numb to it and doesn't reflect on it almost ever. She takes a bite of that burger, and her friends say nothing, because they're in the same boat. They're all on the same boat, and it's sinking. They're going to drown. If we don't make change, we're going to drown.

Bob Harper, Jillian Michaels – personal trainers of the world - save us! Wake us up! Yell at us! Whip us all into shape!

Our tragedy is the wasted potential of people like me – people like everyone in this restaurant - and people like those who sit in front of every one of you, right now. The tragedy is wasted greatness, and it is all around us.

I wrote this book because I believe in you. I may not know you personally, and we may never meet, but regardless of that trivial fact, I believe that you – and every other human being on this planet – were put here to do amazing things. I believe that you have limitless potential and can have the ability to unleash it on this world and make changes that the world needs you to make – changes that you were put on this earth to make. But I do not believe that you can or will unleash that potential until you put your body and mind into a place where they are able to do that. I believe that our unhealthy ways put us into a state that renders us incapable of exercising our true potential. I believe that when the emotions you experience in the morning when you wake up are dependent upon the state your body is in, and if your body is in the wrong state, those emotions and energy levels cannot and will not carry you through the day, doing the things that you were put on this planet to do.

I believe that warmth and happiness can be contagious, and I believe that someone in your life, who you run across today, may *need* you to smile and say hello and help them through a tough time, and I believe that you may not do that when they need you to, if you are not healthy enough to do it. I believe that good health may carry you to smile when you otherwise would not have, to shake a hand you may not have shaken, to send a card you may not have sent, to say "I love you," when you otherwise might not have, and ultimately to spark hope in the life of someone you may not have even acknowledged.

I believe the beauty and progress of this world rest in the collective talents of millions of people, and that those talents go to waste when the millions are stuck in their beds, on their couches, and in their cars, not dreaming because they are living in a fog of obesity and unhealthiness. This world needs you to dream. I need you to dream. Our future and good fortune require that you wake up, ready to face the day, and create what you were put here to create.

I believe you cannot do that if you are not in the mental and physical condition to do so.

I believe, very simply, that you can do more, and I believe that if you do more, and we all do more, we will light a fire that will make this world better than it would have been. I believe it all starts with our physiology, and for me, it all started with the first 30 pounds. I want you to do it too. I believe the world needs you to do it too, and if I can be your partner along that journey and help you just a little, I have written these words.

So let's put a stop to the "norm." Let's get the word out there. Let's talk to people about the weirdness of having sodas all over the place with no place to get a good bottle of Pellegrino. Let's talk to people about going out to lunch every single day at fast food places, and show them how easy it is to cook a few things that taste great and are loaded with vegetables. Let's help people do this together, and flip the world back right side up.

IT NEVER ENDS, SO BE READY

I THINK THAT GREAT people live their lives being grateful, yet unsatisfied. With each milestone I pass, I realize that it never ends. This was just one of them, and there will be many more. When I was younger, I faced financial debt and I always thought, "If I could only get out of debt, I'd be happy." After years, I got out of debt. On that day, I realized that it was just a regular day. Funny, as much as I looked forward to that day, I realized on that day that a whole new flood of productive anxiety was about to come in, including saving for retirement, a wedding someday, and my future children's educations.

So now, I've lost some weight and I've reached another milestone. Just as it was with the debt, I thought that if I could only reach a goal weight, I'd be happy. I'd live life as a healthy, fit, happy person. To some extent, that's actually true. I *am* happier now than I was when I was out of debt. I *am* happier now because I'm healthier. But that same fire is still in me. Now I want more. Now I want to run marathons. Now I want to write books!

I think the point is that no matter how far you swim out to reach the horizon, there's still a horizon out there to swim after. Thank goodness for that, because it's what makes us continue to strive to improve. There will always be something, and that's okay. We never will really feel like we "got there," or at least we won't often stop to do that.

For me, part of "knowing thyself" is knowing that I'll always be striving for something. I can choose to use that to be miserable, or I can use that to my advantage. I'll choose the latter. When I hit a goal, I put a new one out there. I realize the last day of my journey will be the first day of a new one, and I'm always thinking about that next journey.

And so I hope it is this way for you. I hope that you are able to use this advice to lose a few pounds, and to be able to see a new horizon that you couldn't see before due to that weight loss. I hope to have helped you to unlock something in yourself through the weight loss, so that you can unleash potential you may not have even known you had. Remember, life isn't a movie. The credits never roll! Or, when they do, you don't get to read them. So, move onward and upward, and I look forward to hearing what you go on to do next, on the other side of this transformation.

EPILOGUE AND CALL TO ACTION

SO YOU'VE LISTENED TO my story and you've gotten a few tips on how to make your own. Because of one little decision to go see my doctor about weight loss, my life has been sent down a whole new path – a path on which I've written a book, I'm proud of myself, I'm more productive, and I even have anxiety about how much left I have to accomplish. I'm now running, not just walking, toward achieving all of my dreams – and again, it's all because of this diet.

Sometimes the tiniest little decisions to take action can set you off on a whole new course you never knew existed.

Sometimes it's just one little decision to get off the couch just that one day, and that one decision changes everything. Some people live their lives thinking, *if I just hadn't made that one little decision, things would be better.* It goes the other way too. If I just hadn't made that one little decision to leave the office and walk across the street to the doctor's office when I did, you wouldn't be reading this. None of it would have happened.

So, what's your decision? What are you going to do in the ten seconds after you put this book down that might change your life forever? Are you going to set it on the counter and head right back into one of your old patterns? Are you going to set the book down, pick up the phone, and call your doctor to schedule an appointment? The choice is entirely yours. I hope you've already made the right one. I wish you all the best in health and life, and I sincerely thank you for taking this journey with me.

ACKNOWLEDGEMENTS

I WOULD LIKE TO take a moment to show my sincere appreciation and gratitude to the following people and organizations, who without their support and contributions this book would not have been written:

Kim Vitellaro and the incredible, caring, friendly people at Lifescape Medical Associates, Scottsdale, AZ.

Shirley Stoddard, Andrea Stoddard, and Jo Ann McNiel for always telling me I should finally write something, and Ken Stoddard for giving me the work ethic, typing speed, and weekend-morning discipline to actually do it.

Joan Whitlock for always calling me her little Professor even as I climbed into her dog's bed.

Dr. Scott Burrus for being the first person to take my writing of this book seriously, and for sincerely asking to read it. Without that vote of confidence I wouldn't have finished it.

My editors, Kara Hawking, Allison H., and Alison M.

Felicia and Kristen for their incredible research, and Thomas M. for his brilliant cover designs.

Kristin Manvel

Kevin Lustig, Chris Lynne, Steve Marcero

Meghan Malloy for telling me if I didn't write a book soon I'd become old.

The entire leadership team of (and everyone working at) Quicken Loans and the family of companies.

Northcentral University and its outstanding students, faculty, and team members.

Dropbox and Evernote, for making exceptional software that's changing the world and delivering something I've dreamed existed since I first put a Palm Pilot in a cradle to sync it.

Amazon and Amazon KDP for making this all possible for new authors.

ABOUT THE AUTHOR

ERIC STODDARD IS AN author, speaker, executive leader, and the writer of *30 Pounds in 40 Days: One man's weight loss journey with the HCG diet, and a guide to losing weight fast, while creating lasting changes in life, health, motivation, and habits.*

Originally from Rochester, Michigan, Eric holds a bachelor's degree from Michigan State University's James Madison College and Honors College, and a Master's in Business Administration from Northcentral University.

Eric has held professional roles in leadership, training, and finance at organizations including Accenture, Morgan Stanley, Quicken Loans, and Northcentral University.

An Eagle Scout, Eric enjoys outdoor challenges, and has completed successful summits of Mt. Rainier and Mt. Whitney. On any given weekend, you may find Eric climbing the hills of Sedona, Arizona in a Jeep, or motorcycling somewhere in Arizona.

Eric provides live music at restaurants in Scottsdale, Arizona, and has performed music and standup comedy in the Detroit area.

Eric currently lives in Phoenix, Arizona, and can be contacted directly at eric@ericstoddard.com.

THANK YOU, AND LET'S CONNECT!

I'D LIKE TO TAKE a moment to sincerely thank you for reading this, my first book. I'll admit that it wasn't easy for me to put myself out there as a first-time, self-published author, revealing the details of my worst habits, and it means a lot to me that you've taken the time to get as far as this page. I sincerely hope that you got something out of this book, and I'm grateful you've read it. Feel free to contact me personally anytime using the information below.

Write a Review!
If you enjoyed this book, I kindly ask that you take the opportunity to write a review on Amazon.com. If I've provided you some value here, it would mean a great deal to me if you would take a quick moment to write about how this book has helped you.

Email Me!
Please feel free to send me an email at eric@ericstoddard.com. I respond to all email!

Connect on Facebook!
www.facebook.com/ericstoddardauthor

Connect on Twitter:
www.twitter.com/ericstoddard

Subscribe to my Mailing List!
Receive updates on upcoming books! I promise not to bother you often, and you can unsubscribe anytime at the click of a link.
http://www.ericstoddard.com/signup/

REFERENCES

[1] The data show a measurement of 222.5 pounds on 11/14/2013 and a measurement of 193.4 pounds on 12/22/2013, for a precise total of 29.1 pounds of weight loss in 38 days. I ultimately went on to lose even more weight by using the techniques listed in this book.

[2] Smith, J. (2013), Why weight matters in marathons, *Marathon Journal* (3)14, 44-45.

[3] Omichinski, L. (1993), A Paradigm Shift From Weight Loss To Healthy Living. *Obesity & Health*, 7(3), 48.

[4] Kiernan, M., et. al. (2013), Promoting Healthy Weight With "Stability Skills First": A Randomized Trial. *Journal of Consulting and Clinical Psychology*, 81(2), 336-346. doi:10.1037/a0030544

[5] Numeroff, L. J., & Bond, F. (1985), If <u>You Give A Mouse A Cookie.</u> New York: Harper & Row.

[6] Schultz, D.P & Schultz, S. E. (2013), *Theories of Personality* (10th ed.). Belmont, CA: Wadsworth-Cengage Learning.

[7] Heart and Stroke Foundation (2014), *2014 Report on the Health of Canadians*. Ottawa, Ontario, Canada.

[8] ABC News Staff (2012), *100 Million Dieters, $20 Billion: The Weight Loss Industry by the Numbers*. http://abcnews.go.com/Health/100-million-dieters-20-billion-weight-loss-industry/story?id=16297197

[9] Duhigg, C. (2012), The Power of Habit: Why We Do What We Do in Life and Business. New York: Random House.

[10] Ouellette, J.A., & Wood, W. (1998), Habit And Intention In Everyday Life: The Multiple Processes By Which Past Behavior Predicts Future Behavior. Psychological Bulletin, 124, 54–74.

[11] Scott, S. (2002). Fierce Conversations. New York, NY: The Berkley Publishing Group

[12] Howell, J.S. & Shepherd, J.A. (2013). *Behavioral Obligation and Information Avoidance*. Annals of Behavioral Medicine, 45, 258-263.

[13] MensHealth.com, MH Lists (2010). *The 12 Best Smoothie Ingredients.* http://www.menshealth.com/mhlists/best-smoothie-ingredients/index.php?cm_mmc=ABSNL-_-2010_04_02-_-HTML-_-1

[14] Muraven, M. & Collins, R.L. (2005). *Daily Fluctuations in Self-Control Demands and Alcohol Intake.* Psychology of Addictive Behaviors, 19, 140-147; Galliot, M.T. & Baumeister, R.F. (2007). *The Physiology of Willpower: Linking Blood Glucose to Self-Control.* Personality and Social Psychology Review, 11, 303-327.

[15] Sun, T. (2011). *The Art of War: Complete Texts and Commentaries* (T. Cleary, Trans.). Boston, MA and London, England: Shambhala.

[16] U.S. Food and Drug Administration (2013). *Energy "Drinks" and Supplements: Investigations of Adverse Event Reports.* http://www.fda.gov/Food/NewsEvents/ucm328536.htm

[17] Volger, S., et. al. (2013). Changes in eating, physical activity and related behaviors in a primary care-based weight loss intervention. *International Journal of Obesity,* 37S12-S18.

[18] Batra, P., et. al. (2013). Relationship of cravings with weight loss and hunger. Results from a 6-month worksite weight loss intervention. *Appetite,* 691-7.

[19] http://www.hcgdietcouncil.org/history-of-hcg-for-weight-loss/

[20] Simeons, A.T.W. (1954). Pounds and Inches: A New Approach to Obesity.

[21] http://www.doctoroz.com/videos/weight-loss-controversy-hcg-diet-pt-1

[22] Lijesen, G., et. al. (1995). The effect of human chorionic gonadotropin (HCG) in the treatment of obesity by means of the Simeons therapy: a criteria-based meta-analysis. *British Journal Of Clinical Pharmacology,* 40(3), 237-243.

[23] LaBoube, Z. (2013). HCG 2.0: Don't Starve, Eat Smart, and Lose: A Modern Adaption Of The HCG Diet. Irvine: CreateSpace Independent Publishing Platform

[24] The data show a measurement of 222.5 pounds on 11/14/2013 and a measurement of 193.4 pounds on 12/22/2013, for a precise total of 29.1 pounds of weight loss in 38 days.

[25] http://health.howstuffworks.com/wellness/diet-fitness/diets/dangers-hcg-diet.htm

[26] http://health.howstuffworks.com/wellness/diet-fitness/diets/hcg-diet3.htm

27 Fanchin, R., et. al. (2001). Human chorionic gonadotropin: does it affect human endometrial morphology in vivo? *Seminars In Reproductive Medicine,* 19(1), 31-35. *(Full-text unavailable)*

28 http://health.usnews.com/health-news/ diet-fitness/diet/articles/2011/03/14/ hcg-diet-dangers-is-fast-weight-loss-worth-the-risk?page=2

29 http://www.extension.harvard.edu/hub/blog/ extension-blog/how-avoid-harmful-chemicals-your-food

30 Diary, home meals keys to weight loss. (2012). Harvard Women's Health Watch, 20(2), 8.

31 http://well.blogs.nytimes.com/2009/11/04/phys-ed-why-doesnt-exercise-lead-to-weight-loss/

32 Verhoef, S. M., et. al. (2013). Concomitant changes in sleep duration and body weight and body composition during weight loss and 3-mo weight maintenance. *American Journal Of Clinical Nutrition,* 98(1), 25-31.

33 http://running.competitor.com/2013/08/nutrition/ losing-weight-the-right-way-during-marathon-training_1421/3

34 Williams, P. T. (2013). Greater Weight Loss from Running than Walking during a 6.2-yr Prospective Follow-up. *Medicine & Science in Sports & Exercise, 45*(4), 706-713.

[35]   Ann Bolger served as the Director of Residence Life at Michigan State University. She passed away unexpectedly in 2000, and Michigan State University remembers her through the Ann Marie Bolger Memorial Scholarship. To donate, please visit http://education.msu.edu/development/endowed-funds/endowments/bolger.asp

[36]   https://twitter.com/BillPhillips/status/68388767064522752

[37]   http://www.cdc.gov/bloodpressure/facts.htm

[38]   Batra, P., et. al.

[39]   Willett, W. C. (2007). Do grapes and grape juice protect the heart like wine does? *Harvard Heart Letter, 17* (7), 7.

[40]   Chambers, J., & Swanson, V. (2012). Stories of weight management: Factors associated with successful and unsuccessful weight maintenance. *British Journal of Health Psychology, 17*(2), 223-243.

[41]   McKee, H., & Ntoumanis, N. (2014). Developing self-regulation for dietary temptations: intervention effects on physical, self-regulatory and psychological outcomes. *Journal of Behavioral Medicine.*

[42]   Hill, N. (1937) *Think and Grow Rich.* Wilder Publications.

[43] http://www.tonyrobbins.com/resources/pdfs/The-Power-of-Leverage.pdf

[44] www.richroll.com/press/; http://www.mensfitness.com/training/2009-mf-25?page=2

[45] https://www.richroll.com/finding-ultra/

[46] https://medium.com/philosophy-logic/7f838b1fa228

[47] Kearney, M. H., & O'Sullivan, J. (2003). Identity Shifts as Turning Points in Health Behavior Change. *Western Journal Of Nursing Research*, *25*(2), 134-152.

[48] Bovend'eerdt, T., Botell, R., & Wade, D. (2009). Writing SMART rehabilitation goals and achieving goal attainment scaling: a practical guide. *Clinical Rehabilitation*, *23*(4), 352-361.

[49] Conlon, K. E., et. al. (2011). Eyes on the prize: The longitudinal benefits of goal focus on progress toward a weight loss goal. *Journal of Experimental Social Psychology*, 47(4), 853-855.

[50] Dr. Scott Lewis: http://www.drscottlewis.com/visual-reminders-weight-loss-keeping-things-view-will-help-keep-track/

[51] Webber, K. H., et. al. (2010). The effect of a motivational intervention on weight loss is moderated

by level of baseline controlled motivation. *International Journal of Behavioral Nutrition & Physical Activity*, 71-9.

[52] http://well.blogs.nytimes.com/2009/09/03/late-night-eating-linked-to-weight-gain/?_php=true&_type=blogs&_r=00

[53] Gorin, A. A., et. al. (2004). Promoting long-term weight control: does dieting consistency matter? *International Journal of Obesity & Related Metabolic Disorders*, 28(2), 278-281.

[54] http://www.linkedin.com/today/post/article/20140121000245-174077701-productivity-hacks-why-4-a-m-is-the-best-time-to-work

[55] Outland, L., & Stoner-Smith, M. (2013). Promoting Homeostasis To Avoid Rebound Weight Gain In Yo-Yo Dieters. *Internet Journal of Advanced Nursing Practice*, 12(1), 1.

[56] http://choosethinking.com/

[57] http://www.envision-u.com/pr/team.asp

[58] The various weights I post in this book may seem confusing. My official record of weight loss was kept by my scales at home, because this is where I would weigh in sans-clothing and first thing in the morning. Some weigh-ins at the doctor's office were higher because I was clothed and it was already a few hours into the day.

59 http://www.gallup.com/poll/165671/obesity-rate-climbing-2013.aspx

60 http://www.atkins.com/Science/Articles---Library/Nutrition-News/Spring-Clean-Your-Kitchen--Low-carb-tips-for-an-At.aspx; http://www.med-health.net/Dr-Oz-Ultimate-Diet.html

61 http://www.smartertravel.com/blogs/today-in-travel/study-shows-people-happier-before-not-after-vacation.html?id=4403288

62 Phillips, Bill (2003) *Body for Life.* Harper.

63 http://www.doctoroz.com/videos/foods-make-your-belly-flat-vs-fat

64 http://www.webmd.com/diet/features/what-to-do-after-overeating

65 http://www.psychologytoday.com/blog/strive-thrive/201404/four-truths-about-weight-loss-nobody-tells-you

66 Gorin, A., et. al. (2008). Weight loss treatment influences untreated spouses and the home environment: evidence of a ripple effect. *International Journal of Obesity,* 32(11), 1678-1684.

[67] Lieber, C. S. (1991). Perspectives: do alcohol calories count? *American Journal of Clinical Nutrition*, 54(6), 976-982.

[68] https://labeast.com/

[69] Ferriss, T. (2010). The 4-Hour Body: An Uncommon Guide To Rapid Fat-Loss, Incredible Sex, And Becoming Superhuman. New York: Crown Archetype.

[70] Müller, M., Bosy-Westphal, A., & Heymsfield, S. (2010). Is there evidence for a set point that regulates human body weight? *F1000 Medicine Reports*, 259.

[71] Worthy, S. L., et. al. (2010). Demographic and Lifestyle Variables Associated with Obesity. *Health Education Journal*, 69(4), 372-380.

[72] Mandal, B. (2010). Use of Food Labels as a Weight Loss Behavior. *Journal of Consumer Affairs*, 44(3), 516-527.

[73] http://lifehacker.com/281626/ jerry-seinfelds-productivity-secret

[74] www.smartsheet.com

[75] https://www.chopwizard.com/

[76] http://www.gefu.us/

[77] http://www.withings.com/en/bodyanalyzer

[78] http://bustan.net/monitoryourweight

[79] Hebden, L., et. al. (2013). 'TXT2BFiT' a mobile phone-based healthy lifestyle program for preventing unhealthy weight gain in young adults: study protocol for a randomized controlled trial. *Trials, 14*(1), 1-9.

[80] http://realmacsoftware.com/clear

[81] Johnson, F., & Wardle, J. (2011). The association between weight loss and engagement with a web-based food and exercise diary in a commercial weight loss programme: a retrospective analysis. *International Journal of Behavioral Nutrition And Physical Activity, 8*(1), 475.

[82] Mantzios, M., & Wilson, J. C. (2014). Making concrete construals mindful: A novel approach for developing mindfulness and self-compassion to assist weight loss. *Psychology & Health, 29*(4), 422-441. doi:10.1080/0887044 6.2013.863883

[83] Ferriss, T. (2007). *The 4-Hour Workweek.* Crown Publishers, New York.

[84] Allen, D. (2008). Making it all work: winning at the game of work and the business of life. Penguin.

[85] Hülsheger, U. R., Alberts, H. M., Feinholdt, A., & Lang, J. B. (2013). Benefits of mindfulness at work: The role of mindfulness in emotion regulation, emotional exhaustion, and job satisfaction. *Journal Of Applied Psychology*, 98(2), 310-325.

CPSIA information can be obtained
at www.ICGtesting.com
Printed in the USA
LVOW13s0259040118
561757LV00045B/1871/P